Tourette Syndrome:
10 Secrets to a Happier Life

Tourette Treatment Tips

English Edition

Edited by **Michael S. Okun M.D.**

Text copyright © 2017 Michael S. Okun M.D.
michaelokunmd@gmail.com

ISBN: 1542484219
ISBN 13: 9781542484213

Published by Books4Patients

* * *

For discounted bulk orders of the book or any of Dr. Okun's books please contact Books4Patients, LLC at books4patients@gmail.com

* * *

Table of Contents:

* * *

Introduction:

OURETTE SYNDROME (TS) IS AMONG the most mysterious medical curiosities on the planet. The cause(s) of abnormal twitches and movements concurrent with a wide spectrum of behavioral disorders remains completely unknown. We think that TS is inherited and neurodevelopmental; however, there are many critical gaps in our knowledge. The CDC estimates that one in every 362 kids (0.3 percent) has TS and that half of all cases remain undiagnosed. At the Tourette Association of America, experts have estimated it to be even more common at one in 166 kids (0.6 percent). We have yet to discover a single DNA abnormality linking all, or even most, TS cases.

If TS is so common, why is there not more research into cause, treatment and cure? Even though TS, tic disorders and tics are more common than Parkinson's disease, NIH funding for research and discovery pales in comparison to other neurological maladies. Additionally, some TS cases are mild, and many resolve in late adolescence and/or early adulthood, so this resolution may dampen the appetite for research and discovery. The bottom line is that we have a huge TS burden and not enough research into cause, treatment and cure.

The urgency of dealing with TS has never been more pressing. TS threatens our greatest resource: our children. It strikes them in their most formidable years. It hits them when they are in school and when they are developing the philosophies and habits that will serve them over a lifetime. Though it may at a glance appear to the casual observer that TS disappears in adolescence or early adulthood, this is not accurate. The motor and vocal tics do wane in the majority of cases; however, the obsessive compulsive and behavioral features may persist and even escalate. The behavioral features in TS, if left undiagnosed and untreated, will potentially impact quality of life more than motor and vocal tics.

We have taken care of close to 10,000 movement disorder patients at the University of Florida and tens of thousands more with our colleagues in the Southeast Regional Tourette Association of America Center of Excellence (University of South Florida, Emory University, University of Alabama, University of Florida and the University of South Carolina). Over many years, we have come to the disheartening realization that many, if not most, of our patients and families are not aware of the care and education secrets that can help them live happier lives. These practical pearls of wisdom remain secrets, either because they are unknown, or because they are unpracticed. A secret in medicine is not always a pill, procedure or behavioral therapy. A secret can be wisdom on a topic relevant today or any day in the future. We must do a better job to educate TS patients and families. Dean Ornish, a physician from the Preventative Medicine Research Institute, recently said, "An educated patient is empowered; thus more likely to become healthy." We agree with this core principle.

In this book, we have brought together 10 clinical and research experts in TS with the singular goal of assembling 10 secrets on 10 topics we thought could help people on their journey to a happier life with TS. We have organized the book into a simple and easy to digest question and answer format. We envisioned the book to be a cover to cover great read but also an easy reference guide. The chapters are brimming with up-to-date and in many cases cutting-edge strategies and knowledge on TS.

In the first chapter, Ayse Gunduz, a renowned neuroscientist from the University of Florida, reviews the signs of TS and discusses what has and has not been associated with the syndrome. In Chapter 2, Heather Simpson, an occupational therapist also from the University of Florida, reviews all of the important information about accessing and using rehabilitative specialists. In Chapter 3, Douglas Woods, a professor and dean from Marquette University and one of the pioneers of comprehensive behavioral intervention for tics (CBIT), reviews the important and astonishing updates about the usefulness of behavioral TS approaches. In Chapter 4, Lydia Breer, a licensed clinical social worker from Dacula, Georgia with years of experience in TS care, offers top to bottom advice for the use of social workers and counseling therapy. Irene Malaty, a movement disorders neurologist from the University of Florida, in Chapter 5 tells us when to pull the trigger on medications. Irene also reviews commonly used therapies and potential future TS research compounds. In Chapter 6, I will review how and why you may want to make your brain electric with deep brain stimulation (DBS). In Chapter 7, Steve Wu, a pediatric neurologist from Cincinnati Children's Hospital, reviews the latest knowledge and applications of transcranial magnetic and direct current therapies. In Chapter 8, Tanya Murphy, a professor and child psychiatrist from the University of South Florida, brings us up to speed on infectious causes of tics and the syndrome called PANDAS. In Chapter 9, Addie Patterson, a neurologist and fellow-in-residence at the University of Florida, reviews the somewhat surprising facts and potential uses for marijuana therapy. Finally, Kevin McNaught, a well-known scientist and the executive vice president and director of research programs for the Tourette Association of America, ties it all together and tells us where we have been and where we are going in TS research.

On behalf of all the specialists, I offer you our 10 secrets and wish you a happy life with TS. Our core philosophical belief is in patient-centric care. The Tourette patient (not the doctor) should be considered the sun, and our interdisciplinary services should orbit around them.

Michael S. Okun, M.D.
Adelaide Lackner Professor and Chair of Neurology
University of Florida Center for Movement Disorders and Neurorestoration

* * *

CHAPTER 1

Know the Signs

"In complex trains of thought signs are indispensable."
— George Henry Lewes

What is Tourette syndrome?

OURETTE SYNDROME (TS) IS A childhood-onset neurologic
disorder that is caused by abnormalities located in the brain. It
is commonly manifested by multiple phonic (vocal) and motor
(movement) tics. There are also a variety of behavioral issues associated
with TS such as attention deficit hyperactivity disorder, obsessive compulsive disorder and depression[1].

Is Tourette syndrome inherited?

TS is considered a hereditary disorder, and most experts believe that it is
modified by environmental factors. Genetic studies have yet to uncover a

single common causative gene for TS, though there are several candidate genes. Even though in a few cases a causative gene has been implicated, over 90 percent of cases do not have an obvious abnormality present in their DNA. This is why many experts believe that environmental exposures may play a key role in the development of TS[1]. Judith Stern, professor at the University of California, famously said of many diseases, "The genes load the gun, and the environment pulls the trigger."

Who coined the name/eponym Tourette syndrome?

Jean-Martin Charcot, widely considered the founder of modern clinical neurology, coined the name/eponym TS. Charcot's student Georges Albert Gilles de la Tourette provided a description in 1885 of nine patients suffering from a 'malady of tics.' TS had, however, been previously described in cases that were reported by Seprenger and Heinrich in 1498, by Itard in 1825[2], by Trousseau in 1868-1873[3] and by Hughlings Jackson in 1884. Tourette actually recognized the hereditary nature of the syndrome, though in the 100 plus years since his description, it has been commonly mischaracterized by some practitioners as a psychogenic disorder[1, 4].

How variable are the manifestations of Tourette?

There are many variations in the individual clinical manifestations of TS, and there are frequent fluctuations in the severity and frequency of symptoms. It is common for those with TS to also have obsessive compulsive and attention deficit symptoms along with their tics.

The clinical hallmark of TS is sudden, repetitive movements and vocalizations, referred to as tics. These tics have varying degrees of intensity and frequency, and they may be of short or long duration. The course of tics can be unpredictable and is usually variable across patients[1, 4-12].

How are tics classified?

Tics are classified into motor and vocal (phonic) phenomena and can be further sub-classified into simple and complex categories. Simple motor tics involve individual muscles or groups of muscles, whereas complex tics consist of intense, coordinated and sequenced movements, which may in some cases be socially inappropriate. Common simple motor tics include eye blinking, head, neck or limb jerking, sustained mouth opening or shoulder rotation; whereas examples of complex motor tics include touching, hitting, gyrating, bending, echopraxia (imitating actions), copropraxia (gesturing and touching of genitalia), other socially inappropriate behaviors and self-injurious behaviors. Common vocal tics include grunting, squeaking, coughing, sniffing, snorting and throat clearing. Complex vocal tics include meaningful utterances and vocalizations, such as echololia (repeating someone's words), palilalia (repeating one's own words) and coprololia (shouting obscenities or profanities) [1, 4-12].

How common is coprolalia (uncontrollable use of profanity)?

Although coprololia has been characterized on television and in the public as a cardinal feature of TS, it occurs in only 10 to 19 percent of individuals[13-20].

What makes tics worse/better?

It is common for tics to be exacerbated during periods of anticipation, anxiety or fatigue and to be reduced when persons with TS are concentrating on mental or physical tasks. Recent studies have revealed that some tics may persist even during sleep[1, 4-12, 21].

Can tics be suppressed? Does suppression of tics lead to a later rebound worsening?

Tics can be involuntary but can in some cases be voluntarily suppressed. This ability to suppress tics is useful for differentiating TS from other hyperkinetic movement disorders. Although some people feel like their tics get worse temporarily after suppression, most research says that this isn't common[1, 4-12].

What is a premonitory urge?

The onset of both motor and vocal tics frequently is preceded by premonitory urges. These urges are described as a buildup of tension, pressure or energy localized to the tic region or alternatively as a general psychological tension associated with a pressing need to act. Some examples of premonitory urges are muscle tension, nasal stuffiness and dry throat – all preceding the tic. Executing the tic relieves these inner sensations and results in a feeling of relief. Tics have been described by some experts as a "voluntary response to an involuntary sensation." About 90 percent of adults with TS report the occurrence of premonitory urges, whereas 37 percent in the pediatric population report similar sensations. A recent study showed that certain urges could be selectively associated with tics (e.g., physical sensations), and similarly, some urges could be associated with obsessive-compulsive symptoms (e.g., feelings of unease and urgency)[16, 22].

What is self-injurious behavior?

Persons with TS may unintentionally strike themselves as part of a tic or complex of tics. Self- injurious behavior can lead to significant harm, and persons with this issue usually are treated aggressively in an attempt to suppress this behavior[16, 22, 23].

How often do other psychiatric syndromes occur along with Tourette?

The lifetime prevalence of any psychiatric comorbidity among individuals with TS is reported to be approximately 86 percent. Seventy-two percent of TS patients meet the criteria for obsessive-compulsive disorder (OCD) and attention deficit hyperactivity disorder (ADHD). Fifty-eight percent of the TS population was reported to have two or more psychiatric disorders including autism spectral disorders (ASDs), depression, personality disorder, anxiety disorder or self-injurious behavior. These symptoms add to the complex comorbidities associated with TS. These comorbidities can impact quality of life[1, 4-12]..

At what age does Tourette usually manifest? How does it progress?

The clinical course of TS is variable, and the average age at motor tic onset is 5.6 years. Vocal tics have been observed in most cases to follow the onset of motor tics. Studies have revealed that the severity of symptoms peaks at 10.6 years, and following this period of tic intensity, 30 to 50 percent will convert into complete motor tic remission during late adolescence – by age 18. Approximately 30 to 50 percent of TS patients show improvement in symptoms, but in 10 to 20 percent of TS cases, the symptoms fluctuate, persist or worsen. The average age of onset of ADHD has been shown to precede tic symptoms (at approximately 3 years old), whereas the onset for OCD and the peak age of OCD severity occur three to four years following tic onset and peak tic severity. Many ADHD and OCD symptoms persist through adulthood[1, 4-12].

How often does Tourette occur in the population?

The estimated prevalence of TS ranges from three to nine per 1,000 in school-age children. The prevalence is higher in males compared to females with the ratio varying from 2:1 to 4:1. The number of diagnosed cases in the United States is lower among African Americans and Hispanic Americans. This may be related to differences in access to care[1, 4-12].

How disabling are cases of Tourette?

Although TS is not a degenerative disorder, it can be socially crippling, and motor tics may be painful, severe and even life threatening. It has been estimated that five percent of TS patients will be admitted to hospitals each year due to tic-related injuries, self-injurious behavior, uncontrollable violence or suicidal ideation with or without suicide attempts. Such malignant cases have been associated with a greater severity of motor symptoms and the presence of two or more behavioral disorders (comorbidities) [1, 4-12].

❧ Secret #1: The motor and vocal tics in Tourette syndrome are frequently not as disabling as the OCD and behavioral manifestations.

Take Home Points:

- TS is a common disorder and although it has a large genetic component, to date single gene causative mutations have not been common.

- TS has an average age of onset at five to six and peaks in intensity at 10 to 11. In many cases the motor and vocal tics wane in late adolescence and early adulthood.

- TS is one of the most common movement disorders encountered in school systems and clinical practice.

- TS has multiple manifestations including vocal and motor tics, but many of the behavioral manifestations are more disabling (OCD, ADD, etc.).

- Some tics can be simple, and others can be complex and associated with elaborate rituals.

- Stress, anxiety and sleep deprivation can make tics worse.

- Coprolalia (vocal tics involving curse words) is a relatively uncommon manifestation.

- Tics are often associated with premonitory urges. Once a person with TS recognizes a premonitory urge, the performance of the tic usually reduces anxiety.

- Tics and other TS symptoms can in many cases be very disabling.

*Quotes and sections of this chapter were provided with special written permission from the publisher of a recent review article, Springer. Gunduz, A., Okun, M.S., A Review and Update on Tourette Syndrome: Where Is the Field Headed? Curr Neurol Neurosci Rep. 2016 Apr; 16(4):37. doi: 10.1007/s11910-016-0633-x. Review. PubMed PMID: 26936259.

* * *

CHAPTER 2:

Know How to Access Rehabilitative Therapies

"I'm addicted to success. Thankfully, there's no rehab for success."
— Lil Wayne

Who are the rehabilitation specialists who may be most helpful in treating Tourette syndrome?

PSYCHOLOGY, PSYCHIATRY AND NEUROLOGY HAVE traditionally been the primary professions engaged by the health care system in the treatment of Tourette syndrome (TS) and tic disorders. Recently, other health care professionals have teamed with these three disciplines to help enhance the well-being and quality of life for children and adults with tic disorders. Interdisciplinary clinics are increasingly being created to capitalize on the benefits of additional professionals who can contribute to enhancing the quality and diversity of care. The main three rehabilitation professions that may play a role in helping persons with TS include occupational therapy, physical therapy and speech-language pathology[24-27].

Why consult occupational, physical and speech-language pathology specialists for the treatment of Tourette syndrome?

People living with TS have an increased likelihood of comorbid conditions (having more than one diagnoses or condition), and both the TS and comorbidity can affect daily life. Occupational therapy, physical therapy and speech-language pathology treat both the TS motor and vocal tics but also address the comorbid conditions that can be more limiting and impactful on daily life. Some of the most common comorbid conditions include Attention Deficit Hyperactivity Disorder (ADHD), Obsessive-Compulsive Disorder (OCD) and/or anxiety. Research has shown that approximately 86 percent of TS patients have a co-occurring neurobehavioral (relating to the nervous system and behavior) condition that impedes daily activities. Management of these comorbid conditions has been shown to lead to an increased quality of life, and this is the best rationale to bring in occupational therapy, physical therapy, and speech-language pathology. Unfortunately, however, these comorbid conditions are frequently placed on hold, as treatment of the motor and vocal tics may be overemphasized. Despite the associated and comorbid conditions often being the primary cause of limitation, they are commonly ignored. When left untreated, these conditions can indirectly impact tics and lead to a worsening of the overall TS[13-15, 17, 23-30].

How available are rehabilitative services for Tourette Syndrome?

Well-trained and thoroughly educated providers to address TS symptoms and associated conditions are not widely available. Families may therefore be forced to travel long distances for treatment or may actually avoid appropriate treatment. Interestingly, rehabilitation services tend to be more accessible and more frequently available than physician care, even in rural communities. These services may also be available and embedded within the school system.

What is Occupational Therapy?

Occupational Therapy (OT): OT is defined as "the therapeutic use of everyday life activities (occupations) with individuals or groups for the purpose of enhancing or enabling participation in roles, habits, and routines in home, school, the workplace, the community, and in other settings." This definition of OT translates into helping others achieve independence in activities they wish to perform and activities that will result in increased enjoyment in their life. Occupational therapists can also now be certified to implement and treat using the Comprehensive Behavioral Intervention for Tics (CBIT) program as recognized by the Behavior Therapy Institute (BTI) and the Tourette Association of America[25]. We will review the use of OT therapists in CBIT in Chapter 3.

What is Physical Therapy?

Physical Therapy (PT): PT is defined as a rehabilitative "profession with an established theoretical and scientific base and with widespread clinical applications in the restoration, maintenance, and promotion of optimal physical function." Physical therapy enables people to successfully engage in the world around them by addressing physical function and mobility[26].

What is Speech-Language Pathology (SLP)?

Speech-Language Pathology (SLP): SLP is defined as therapists who "work to prevent, assess, diagnose, and treat speech, language, social communication, cognitive-communication, and swallowing disorders in both children and adults[27]." Speech-language pathology enables people to have more effective communication and swallowing skills in all aspects of daily life. The terms speech-language pathologist and speech therapists (ST) will be used interchangeably for the purposes of this chapter.

What is Sensory Integration Dysfunction?

"My child does not like tags in her clothes. I am a picky eater. I am hypersensitive to sounds."

Sensory integration (SI) is a normal, neurological process that shapes who we are as humans. Sensory integration dysfunction is based on a theory from Jean Ayers, who hypothesized that brain function and how we interpret the sensory environment around us actually shapes our human behavior. For example, how we interpret touch from others, the feeling of tags in our clothes or the feeling we get when being tickled can be perceived as offensive and lead to increased awareness or defensiveness[29].

How can Sensory Integration Dysfunction affect Tourette Syndrome?

SI has been widely recognized as a problem in the Tourette community but is rarely treated effectively. The occupational therapist should try to understand the exact nature of SI difficulties in both adults and children with TS by utilizing a variety of testing and treatment strategies. According to the Tourette Association of America,[31, 32] many people with tic disorders can have sensory integration difficulties including but not limited to:

- Difficulty with sitting still in class (other than related to tics)

- Hypersensitivity to sounds, sights or textures

- Overstimulation in busy environments

What is a sensory diet and how can it help Tourette?

To address SI concerns, an occupational therapist may introduce you to a "sensory diet." A "sensory diet" is a personalized, structured program that is designed to appropriately integrate and manage your sensory needs and to decrease the adverse sensory responses throughout the day. If picky eating habits (e.g. eating unhealthy foods) arise due to sensory integration difficulties, there are occupational therapists who have received a specialty certification and are trained in the management of increasing a child's chances to have a healthy diet. An occupational therapist who is familiar with the sensory system and the sensory integration approach would be a valuable team member if sensory dysfunction concerns are uncovered[33].

What is executive dysfunction and why is it important in Tourette syndrome?

"My child always loses his homework." "My loved one is disorganized and messy."

Executive function is defined as "self-regulatory behaviors necessary to select and sustain actions and to guide behavior within the context of goals or rules[34]." Executive functions are needed to engage in higher order thinking and processing in order to regulate behaviors and actions but also to plan activities and to complete goal-oriented activities. The Tourette Association of American recognizes that executive dysfunction is a common comorbid condition in those suffering from TS. Some examples of executive dysfunction in TS include[31, 32]:

- Difficulty with organization

- Difficulty with making decisions

- Difficulty with problem-solving

- Difficulty with time management

- Difficulty with inhibition

- Difficulty with emotional control

What causes executive dysfunction and is it treatable?

When the prefrontal cortex (one of the regions of the brain important for executive function) is not working appropriately, functional limitations can occur throughout the day that can create difficulty at school for children and problems at work for adults. Speech and occupational therapists have had long standing success in improving executive dysfunction. Research studies have developed treatment strategies that have been shown to be effective in remediating and retraining the thinking process while also improving processing speed to manage problem solving capabilities. Speech and occupational therapists can introduce compensatory strategies to increase success in various environments. Seeking rehabilitation services to support and train executive functions can be a promising approach for increasing success and decreasing frustration with daily activities[33].

Do attention difficulties occur in Tourette syndrome and how do they impact the person with Tourette?

"My child cannot sit still during school.""My wife does not seem to focus enough and listen."

Attention Deficit Hyperactivity Disorder (ADHD) and Attention Deficit Disorder (ADD) are common associated conditions that occur with TS. Current research has demonstrated that these conditions occur in as many as 60 percent of those affected by TS[28]. Attention difficulties are considered by many experts to be a part of the executive dysfunction. Attention limitations impact quality of life. Limited ability to attend to a task can be related to many factors including:

- Sensory integration difficulties

- The tics themselves and the need to suppress or manage tics

- Genetic factors related to ADHD

Difficulty paying attention leads to functional limitations such as:

- Difficulty in school

- Difficulty with following directions

- "Getting in trouble"

- Problems with structured activities[13-15, 17, 23, 28, 30, 35]

Are there training techniques that can be used to improve attention?

Training for improved attention has been closely linked to the executive function training methods that therapists have employed to increase self-awareness and improve self-control strategies. Occupational therapists utilize tools such as fidgets (fidget rings, gear ties) or alternative seating (special bouncy seats for kids) that have been shown to be effective in increasing attention. Speech therapists can be trained to promote improvement in the higher levels of attention required for complex situations such as engaging in conversation. Management of attentional limitations can be addressed by using rehabilitative services such as speech and occupational therapy. Many techniques can help with training the higher level cognitive functions required to improve the ability to attend to daily tasks[27, 33].

Do Tourette syndrome patients have impaired arousal and stress management?

"My loved one gets angry very quickly," or "My child seems to make decisions without thinking."

Adults and children with Tourette syndrome frequently have difficulty controlling anger and may also have associated trouble controlling impulsivity (acting in a situation where action or engagement may not be appropriate). Anger and impulse control may also be related to executive dysfunction and poor emotional regulation. It has been thought that these issues may be the result of dysfunction in regions of the brain known to be affected in TS (basal ganglia and frontal cortex)[36]. Many times, an inability to control one's frustration can lead to increased behavioral difficulties as well as impair social relations. TS patients often act without thinking[37]. Chang, Liang, Wang, Li, Ko & Hsu (2008) showed that the more severe the tics, the more aggression and externalizing behavior problems existed. TS patients may act out and can have aggressive thoughts and actions[37].

Can arousal and stress management be taught?

Occupational therapists can assist psychology and mental health counselors in teaching arousal and stress management. Addressing these issues is helpful in teaching control of anger and impulse issues. There are stress management techniques and stress awareness programs that when employed can be very helpful. Programs such as How Does Your Engine Run[*] and the Child & Parent Resource Institute's The Brake Shop have been frequently utilized to teach increased awareness of self-arousal and prevent abnormal responses to unwanted actions. In addition to training arousal level self-awareness, there has been much research that has revealed the benefits of stress management in management of both stress and arousal states. Managing stress and impaired arousal can have an indirect effect on tics. For example, stress management programs, such as mindfulness programs, have been shown to decrease tic frequency[38].

What social and pragmatic skills can be useful in treating Tourette syndrome?

"My loved one does not have any friends." "My son gets bullied a lot."
The Tourette Association of America has recognized that children and adults with TS might have difficulty with reading social cues and with interacting with others[39]. Common issues include difficulty in knowing what to say, how to effectively communicate, how to appropriately react, how to use appropriate body language (or touch) and how to modulate volume of voice[40]. These difficulties can be related to many factors including the tics themselves, the comorbid conditions (such as Autism

Spectrum Disorder or Social Communication Disorder) or the impaired peer interactions. It is unfortunate but common that many school-aged children with tics are victims of bullying and often shy away from social situations. Adults with tics may not feel comfortable with introducing themselves in new settings, and later in adolescence may have trouble initiating dating. Occupational therapy and speech therapy can be useful in helping both children and adults develop strategies to increase success. Some skill set training strategies might include but are not limited to:

- Reading social cues

- Utilizing appropriate language and communication skills

- Teaching conversation skills

- Social skills groups

- Managing bullying

Addressing bowel and bladder dysfunction in Tourette

"My child still wets the bed at night," or "My loved one suffers from constipation."
Pelvic health physical therapy is one of the latest and trending successful treatment methods in adults with incontinence or pelvic dysfunction[41]. There is a growing trend favoring the use of pediatric physical therapy to manage pelvic health issues such as bedwetting or constipation. Coming & Comings (1987) reported that children with TS had a difference in bowel and bladder control related to a delay in toilet training and to an increase in bedwetting when compared to those without tic disorders[42]. Research has also revealed that children with ADHD have a higher instance of incontinence[43]. Having difficulties with pelvic floor dysfunction can be painful (e.g. constipation) or limiting socially (e.g. inability of a child to have sleep-over because of bed wetting). Pelvic floor physical therapy has been shown to be an effective non-pharmacologic treatment in managing these symptoms that can be debilitating and limiting in quality of life for both children and adults with TS[41].

Can handwriting skills (dysgraphia) be improved in Tourette?

"I cannot read my loved one's handwriting." "My child takes twice as long to complete handwriting homework."
Handwriting is a critical skill that is needed for school success despite the growing trend for children to use electronic devices. Tics that physically occur with handwriting (such as rewriting words, jerking of an arm or eye blinking) can render writing difficult, but in addition to the tics, the actual task of handwriting can be cumbersome. Handwriting involves many components that can contribute to success including visual motor skills, fine motor skills and oculomotor skills. It is important to have an occupational therapist evaluate all components of handwriting as well as address fatigue that may result from writing, illegibility and the writing speed. Addressing handwriting concerns in early elementary school can be more effective than waiting until it becomes an increased concern and the workload increases in school.

Do sleep difficulties worsen Tourette?

"My child is on medication to help him fall asleep at night." "My tics are worse right before bed."
According to the National Sleep Foundation, adults require seven to nine hours of sleep a night, teenagers require eight to 10 hours and children need the most sleep at nine to 11 hours. Numerous studies have revealed that only 15 percent of teenagers get the recommended amount of sleep, and we suspect those with TS get even less quality sleep[44-46]. Studies have shown that both adults and children with TS have difficulties staying asleep at night, have abnormal movements in sleep and difficulties falling asleep[44-46]. Poor sleep results in worsened motor and vocal tics the following day. Additionally, cognitive tasks and control of emotion can be affected in those with TS.

Working with an occupational therapist, evidence-based "sleep hygiene" strategies can be employed. Occupational therapists can assess your sleep patterns and formulate recommendations as well as refer for sleep studies.

What are some tips for helping Tourette patients get jobs?

"My loved one has difficulty with keeping a job." "I am concerned about my teenager ever having the ability to get a job."

The Tourette Syndrome Impact Survey showed that adolescents had concerns about gaining future employment (2013)[47]. Occasionally, tics and comorbid conditions can interfere with performance of the tasks that are needed to sustain meaningful employment. Occupational therapy, speech therapy and the Centers for Independent Living, along with your state's Vocational Rehabilitation can help to address the issue of job finding and job security. Developing strategies for work success and on-the-job training can help a TS patient succeed in the workforce. An occupational therapist is an expert in determining how to modify and adapt the work environment to increase success in job-related duties. All rehabilitation therapists inclusive of physical therapy, occupational therapy and speech and language pathology are trained to have a deep understanding of the Americans with Disabilities Act (ADA). This understanding is critical as therapists can help ensure regulations are enforced and implemented in your workplace.

Can speech dysfluency and reading comprehension difficulties in Tourette be addressed?

"My husband frequently gets stuck on his words." "My child seems to have trouble reading."

In a 2005 study by De Nil, Sasisekharan, Pascal, Lieshout, & Sandor, children with TS reported perceived difficulties in speech related tasks including stuttering and reading[48]. Learning disabilities as a comorbid condition to TS can be a limiting factor in school success. As many as 22 percent of children with TS have been documented to have a learning disability[28]. Reading and also interpreting information on a page can be difficult. Reading and understanding words as well as grammar related to writing skills can be a large part of learning difficulties[40]. In addition, reading assignments and testing sessions can be a time when frustration and stress worsen tics. Speech therapists are highly trained in teaching strategies to increase success with reading comprehension. Management may include formulating thoughts and learning to correctly vocalize. Speech therapists can also test for dyslexia and provide evidence-based treatment programs for it. In addition to reading difficulties, speech or language dysfluency (problems with flow of speech) can result in stammering over words or stuttering. Approximately seven percent of TS patients have experienced a stutter that impacts verbal skills[28]. Stuttering can also be a tic and may be addressed with the Comprehensive Behavioral Intervention for Tics (CBIT) program which will be discussed in Chapter 3. Stuttering could also be a developmental dysfluency, and treatment of each type of stuttering or tic could be variable[49]. A thorough evaluation should be able to separate a stutter from a tic.

Can rehabilitation therapists address problems with coordination, postural instability, pain and weakness in Tourette?

"My child appears clumsy and falls a lot." "I just like to sit around and play video games all day."

Tics can have indirect effects on physical activity because they may create pain, lead to fatigue or impair motion. Decreased physical activity, such as increased time with video games or television and increased homework loads, results in less physical exercise. Physical therapists can address all the gross motor issues that may accompany TS. If your child demonstrates difficulties with ball skills, appears clumsy or even uncoordinated, these issues can all be addressed. For example, one TS study revealed problems with balance when the eyes were closed. Therefore, it suggests potential postural stability testing was useful for those with gross motor concerns[50]. Creation of a home exercise program for core strengthening and postural improvements has the potential to help. Establishing a regular exercise routine can also be very helpful. Nixon, Glazebrook, Hollis & Jackson (2014) reported that moderate level exercise had immediate positive impact on tics[51]. Also, many studies have collectively demonstrated that adults and children with TS were more likely to suffer from muscle, bone and joint discomfort[28]. Physical therapists can also help to map a strategy for pain management. Pain may be associated with TS and may occur from injury or stress during a movement.

How can assistive technologies be used to improve Tourette?

"I don't have the resources to help my child succeed." "I know there have to be technology resources to help my loved one, but I just do not know where to find them."

The Technology-Related Assistance Act of 1998 defined the term "assistive technology" as "a device and a service which is any item, piece of equipment, or product system, whether acquired commercially, modified, or customized, that is used to increase, maintain, or improve the functional capabilities of individuals with disabilities[52]." TS patients who may suffer from functional limitations such as issues with handwriting, typing, utensil use or physical movements could benefit from an assistive technology assessment through either occupational or speech therapy. Assistive technology options include tools such as voice recording pens, applications to assist with handwriting, organizational tools, fidgets, communications applications, alternative seating and physical modification devices.

How do I get plugged in with rehabilitative services for Tourette?

- **Step 1:** Do your research.

  o If any of the associated/comorbid conditions above sound familiar, read about them. Try to better understand how you or your loved one may be influenced by TS.

o Understand what service(s) you may be looking for and what possible options may be in your area.

- **Step 2:** Talk with your medical professional.

  o Share your concerns and ask your physician to complete a screening and to refer to the appropriate resources.

    - Your physician might recommend a neuropsychological assessment to determine what associated/comorbid conditions are present prior to referring. A neuropsychological assessment is a comprehensive battery of testing that will assess cognitive, visual and various other mental functioning skills.

  o Discuss your desire with your doctor to employ a multi-disciplinary approach. The Tourette Association of America has many resources available. The website is www.tourette.org.

- **Step 3:** Ask for a referral to appropriately screen for each of your concerns.

  o If your physician or medical professional agrees that a referral to a rehab service is warranted, they can facilitate an appointment with an outpatient clinic providing those services.

  o Ask your physician if they have a preferred clinic or rehabilitation therapist with which they work or collaborate well.

  o If your physician is not aware of a specific clinic or cannot recommend a therapist by name, search the following websites for registered and licensed professionals:

    - Speech-language pathologists: http://asha.org/

    - Occupational therapists: Individual State Department websites

    - Physical therapists: http://www.apta.org/

o The Tourette Association of America provides an allied health professional list of providers in different disciplines that have registered as accepting TS patients.

How do I obtain school accommodations for Tourette?

If you are seeking help for your child in public school and require accommodations related to school performance and school success, it is very important to reach out to your rehabilitation team and/or physician. Most professionals will be willing to write a letter requesting a 504 plan or an Individualized Education Plan (IEP) for appropriate accommodations at school. Once a meeting has taken place and determination reached by the school through the use of an IEP/504 plan, it can be decided if your child will receive rehabilitative services in the school system. In many circumstances, occupational, physical or speech therapy can be provided within the school system if tasks are deemed to be interfering with the education process and goals.

?❧ Secret #2: Rehabilitative Tourette syndrome therapies can be as powerful as medicines and behavioral therapies.

Take Home Points:

- Rehabilitative specialists can provide meaningful input and strategies for the management of TS. These specialties include occupational therapy, physical therapy and speech and language therapy.

- Recognizing that TS is associated with other issues beyond the motor and vocal tics will help to more effectively address the disorder.

- Identifying and addressing sensory integration dysfunction can improve quality of life and lessen the disability associated with TS.

- Evaluating for the potential of executive dysfunction can help to focus the treatment plan and improve outcomes.

- Make sure if there are difficulties in school that an Individualized Education Plan (IEP) is constructed and implemented.

- If there are communication issues, involve a speech and language therapist as early as possible.

- Developing social skills often requires occupational and speech therapists to develop a plan to address deficiencies.

- Stress management strategies will make a huge difference in TS outcomes.

- Sleep can be affected by TS. If TS patients do not get a good night's sleep, they will likely not have a productive next day.

- Know where the resources are for assisting job training, placement and work modifications.

* * *

CHAPTER 3:

Know When to Employ Cognitive Behavioral Intervention Therapy and Habit Reversal Strategies

"Quality is not an act, it is a habit."

— Aristotle

A T FIRST GLANCE, BEHAVIORAL TREATMENTS can be confusing. Questions are often asked such as: "If a behavioral treatment works, does that mean that my child's problem isn't a real illness but just bad *behavior*? If I learn to manage my tics through a behavioral treatment, does that mean that tics were learned? Did I do something that caused my child to have tics?"

These questions are understandable but based on a misunderstanding of behavior therapy and its purpose. Before describing behavioral treatments for tics, it is worth talking about what causes our behavior and what causes our behavior to differ from moment to moment and person to person.

What defines human behavior?

Everything we do is behavior. We breathe, think, feel, talk and move. But what causes us to do these things? Our behavior is caused by– or "a function of"– two things that work with each other. These two things, our brain and our environment, play an important role in the creation of both normal and abnormal behavior. Let us start with the brain.

Our brain's main role is to keep us alive. It keeps us alive, of course, by doing things like maintaining our breathing, heartbeat and body temperature and by giving us the ability to move in a coordinated, smooth fashion. However, it also keeps us alive in other ways. Through evolution, our brains developed the ability to help survive in different environments. As new structures in the brain evolved, our ability to learn from successes and mistakes increased. We developed the capacity to repeat actions that brought pleasure or provided relief, to avoid painful or threatening situations and to hold back impulses to do things that ultimately were not in our best interest. The evolution of the brain offered humans the ability to enter and thrive in many different environments.

However, the brain alone does not cause behavior. It takes "two to tango" – so the saying goes. We also need the environment in which the brain exists in order to actually produce behavior. Our environment delivers the pleasurable consequences the brain decides it would like to have more of. The environment facilitates the pain or discomfort that our brain learns to avoid or escape from. It delivers the things that make it worth setting aside our immediate impulses. Most importantly, our environment and the experiences we have in those environments change our brain. As a result, environment and experiences impact our thinking, feeling and acting over time.

What is neuroplasticity and why is it important?

The concept of neuroplasticity, long accepted in neuroscience, is the idea that our brain is not set in stone. How it operates is affected greatly through interactions with our environment. Through these interactions, our brain can sharpen existing skills or acquire new ones. Neural pathways get stronger or weaker depending on experiences we have with our environment. It is this fact that allows stroke victims to regain the ability to speak or walk through therapies like physical rehabilitation. It is what enables children to learn to ride bicycles or to easily learn a new language. It is what allows professional athletes to be the best at their sport. It is also a core principle behind behavior therapy.

What is the basis for behavior therapy?

Behavior therapy is based on two ideas. The first is that behavior is a result of both brain and environment. If the brain has not developed as it should, behavior will likely be abnormal. Likewise, even if the brain is perfectly normal, behavior can be abnormal if the environment is not normal. Raise a child with a perfectly normal brain in an environment that does not reward or encourage learning – or fail to expose that child to adequate educational material – and that child will likely not grow up with an average IQ.

The second idea behind behavior therapy is that behavior can be changed by changing the environment. If brain abnormalities lead to abnormal behaviors, changes in the environment can help correct the brain's abnormalities or teach the person to cope with or control the abnormal behavior more effectively. Likewise, if abnormal environments lead to abnormal behaviors, behavior therapy can correct the environment and allow the normal brain to work as it should.

In tic disorders, behavior therapy does the former. It is well understood that tic disorders are the result of subtle abnormalities in the brain. So regardless of what happened in their past, children with these brain abnormalities will develop tics. However, tics are behavior, and when behavior happens, the environment will start controlling them. As a result, certain settings will trigger tics, and when tics result in pleasure or relief, the brain will want to repeat them. In other words, tics are caused by abnormal brain functioning that limits the ability to inhibit movements. However, after the tics appear they become more frequent, intense and varied, and they are modulated by the environment.

What is the purpose of behavior therapy?

The purpose of behavior therapy is two-fold. First, behavior therapy changes the environment so tics do not lead to pleasurable outcomes or produce relief. This is important because such consequences are likely to make tics stronger. Behavior therapy also changes situations that trigger tics. Behavior therapy changes the brain as the brain learns that tics do not result in anything useful for the person. Second, behavior therapy teaches the person with tics to better inhibit unwanted movements, and by doing so attempts to build a new neural pathway to correct the brain abnormality that originally caused the tics. The most common form of behavior therapy for tics is known as the Comprehensive Behavioral Intervention for Tics or CBIT. ("see-bit")[53-56].

What is CBIT therapy?

CBIT is a non-drug strategy for managing tics. Children with TS and their families learn CBIT with the help of a therapist trained in the procedure. Although CBIT sounds like a common form of therapy called CBT (cognitive-behavior therapy), they are different. CBIT is a specialized form of CBT. A therapist may know how to do CBT, but it does not mean they know how to do CBIT. Typically CBIT is taught to a patient in about eight sessions. In the first session, the therapist will get to know more about the tics and will give the patient and his or her family information about TS. In later sessions, the therapist will work with the family to determine how the environment is making the tics increase and will provide specific suggestions for changing the environment in order to better manage tics. The therapist will also teach the patient specific tic-control strategies. During CBIT, the therapist may seem more like a coach than a therapist, because in a way they are. As we tell therapists when we train them in CBIT, "The goal of CBIT is to make the patient so good at managing their own tics that they no longer need your help." CBIT involves many elements that are put together in a way to help the patient learn to effectively manage tics.

What are function-based assessments and interventions?

Tics can be heavily influenced by environmental surroundings. When a tic is reliably influenced by a particular person, place or thing, the tic is said to be a *function* of the environment. Part of CBIT is to determine the environmental factors that worsen tics for a patient. This process is called functional assessment. In functional assessment, the therapist and patient (and parent, if the patient is a child) review situations during which tics occur more frequently or more intensely than usual. When tics occur more frequently or intensely than usual, it is likely that something in the environment is triggering or reinforcing them.

During the functional assessment, the therapist looks for antecedents and consequences to tics. Antecedents are things in the environment that trigger tics, and consequences are reactions to tics that may reinforce them. In performing the functional assessment, the therapist is not looking for the cause of tics (since tics are biological) but the things in the environment that will make tics worse.

For example, assume the functional assessment interview tells us that 13-year-old Sullivan's tics are worse at night, right before he goes to bed. As we talk with Sullivan and his parents, we find that every night before bed, Sullivan starts to worry about the next school day. When he worries, he gets anxious and his tics increase. When he tics, his parents let him stay up until his tics calm down. While he is waiting he gets to watch television with his parents instead of going to bed. In this case, the therapist might assume that Sullivan's tics are both a function of anxiety (i.e., Sullivan tics more when he is anxious) and also a function of getting to watch television with his parents (i.e., when Sullivan tics a lot at night, he gets to stay up late and watch television).

After a therapist has identified the various environmental factors that may trigger and reinforce tics, the therapist develops function-based interventions for the patient and his or her family. A function-based intervention is a simple strategy or skill the patient and/or family can use to better manage the tics. A function-based intervention is directly linked to what was learned during the functional assessment.

Back to our example, Sullivan's tics were worse when he was anxious and were likely being reinforced by being allowed to stay up late and watch television. As a function-based intervention, a therapist would likely teach Sullivan a relaxation technique he could use when he starts to get anxious, and this technique would help reduce his tics. The therapist may also work with Sullivan to determine the source of his worries about school and work with him to view school as more manageable. Collectively, this approach should also reduce his anxiety and his tics. The therapist in this case would also be likely to recommend that Sullivan's parents no longer allow him to stay up late and watch television until his tics diminish. Rather, they should set a fixed bedtime and have him practice the relaxation strategies before going to bed.

The aforementioned example is one of the many ways in which the environment can impact tics and one of the many environmental change strategies a therapist may recommend. Sometimes the patient is taught a skill to more effectively change his or her environment (e.g. relaxation). Sometimes the parent or significant other is asked to do something differently. Sometimes school personnel are asked to help by setting up the classroom in a way that makes tics less likely to happen, by educating the patient's peers about tics so the peers do not react to the tics or by reacting to tics differently themselves. All of this is performed with the goal of more effective tic management.

Although function-based interventions can sometimes seem obvious, parents should obtain advice from a CBIT expert when seeking a functional assessment and implementing function-based interventions[53-56].

What is habit reversal training (HRT)?

A second key element of CBIT is habit reversal training (HRT). HRT involves teaching the patient to control his or her tics in a gradual fashion. Most people can actually sense their tics are about to happen. They experience an unpleasant sensation right before the tic occurs. Sometimes this is described as a pressure, urge or itch. In scientific terms, it is called a premonitory urge, and it is a signal the tic is about to occur.

People with tics also notice that the urge will disappear temporarily, right after the tic(s). In HRT, the person with tics is made more aware of this urge, taught to do a tic-preventing exercise whenever the urge occurs and to continue this exercise until the urge fades away on its own. This process is called habituation. By repeatedly practicing the exercise when the urge is present, the person with tics retrains his or her brain to more effectively inhibit the unwanted movements.

HRT involves three procedures: awareness training, competing response training and social support. For each of the patient's tics, the procedures that make up HRT are practiced with the patient. In CBIT, the therapist typically performs HRT on one tic per week. Sometimes all of the patient's tics are treated, and sometimes only the patient's most bothersome tics are addressed, depending on the patient's preference[57].

What is awareness training?

HRT begins with awareness training. The process of making a patient more aware of his or her tics is accomplished through a therapist and patient working together to develop a detailed description of the tic. The therapist encourages the patient to describe the movements involved in the tic as well as the sensations he or she experiences during the tic(s). After developing a thorough description, the patient practices "catching" the tics as they happen during a treatment session. The therapist asks the patient to raise a finger every time the patient notices him or herself performing the tic that is being targeted. As the therapist and patient talk, the therapist watches the patient to make sure he or she is accurately detecting the tics. If the patient correctly notices the tic and raises his or her finger, the therapist praises the patient briefly before returning to the conversation. If the patient does the tic without acknowledging it, the therapist points this out to the patient. The process continues until the patient accurately detects approximately 80 percent of his or her tics. At this point, the therapist encourages the patient to detect the tics even earlier – when the premonitory urge appears but prior to the tic occurrence. The therapist and patient continue to talk, and the patient is encouraged to raise a finger each time the urge appears. The therapist praises the patient for accurately detecting the urge, but if the patient tics without raising his or her finger, the therapist encourages the patient to do so when the urge first appears. This process continues until the patient regularly notices the urge.

What is competing response training?

After the patient has become more aware of his or her tic, the therapist and patient begin competing response training. A competing response is a behavior the patient performs when he or she notices the tic has occurred or when the premonitory urge is present. When the urge is present or the tic has occurred, the patient should immediately perform the competing response for one minute or until the urge goes away (whichever takes longer). In general, a competing response is an action the patient performs that (a) prevents the tic from occurring, (b) can be held for a minute or until the urge goes away and (c) is less noticeable than the tic it is being used to combat.

Competing response training begins with the therapist describing what makes a good competing response. Next, the therapist asks the patient to select a competing response. After a good competing response is chosen, the therapist demonstrates how and when it should be performed. The therapist practices the competing response with the patient and asks the patient to perform the competing response when the tic happens or when the urge to tic occurs. If the patient performs the competing response correctly in session, the therapist praises the patient. If the patient tics in session but forgets to do the competing response, the therapist will prompt the patient. This procedure continues until the patient reliably uses the competing response in session.

After the patient has shown he or she can perform the competing response correctly, the patient is sent home with an assignment of performing the competing response for the tic on which he or she is working. The patient is asked to perform the competing response whenever the target tic or related premonitory urge occurs. Patients often feel they are performing the competing response "all the time" when first starting work on a tic, but patients quickly notice the tic fades with repeated practice of the competing response.

Why is social support needed for CBIT?

To encourage the correct use of the competing response, a social support component is often added to HRT. Social support is not simply being a supportive person in the patient's life. Rather in HRT, the social support person has two specific jobs. First, if the patient is seen doing the tic but not performing the competing response, the support person is asked to gently remind the person by saying something such as "don't forget to do your exercises." Second, if the patient is seen performing the competing response correctly, the support person is asked to praise the patient by saying something such as "nice job doing your exercises." CBIT therapists often encourage the support person to refrain from praising the patient for 'not ticing.' In CBIT, the patient learns that he or she does not really control whether or not the tics happen but does have control over whether or not the competing response is used. For this reason, support persons are encouraged to praise and prompt the correct use of the competing response rather than praise or punish the patient for tic.

What are other important elements of CBIT?

Even though function-based interventions and HRT are the primary components of CBIT, CBIT also has other parts including education about tics, relaxation training and activities performed to enhance the patient's motivation for treatment. Each of these components is described below.

Psychoeducation. Patients often come to therapy with little information about their disorder. Part of learning to manage tics is to strive to understand tics. CBIT therapists spend time in the first one or two sessions administering common information about tics. This often results in the patient feeling more positive about his or her condition and offers some understanding as to how a disorder that seems so uncontrollable can be managed effectively.

Relaxation Training. Most people with tics recognize that tics worsen when feeling stressed or anxious. Whether or not anxiety or stress actually makes tics worse remains debatable, but what is clear is that when a person is stressed, tics become harder to control. For this reason, CBIT trains patients to relax in stressful situations, often making their tics easier to manage. In CBIT, relaxation training involves two parts. First, the patient is taught a relaxed style of breathing called diaphragmatic breathing. Second, he or she is taught to relax his or her body through tensing and relaxing specific muscle groups. After the patient has learned these skills in therapy, he or she is asked to practice these relaxation techniques at home.

Motivation. Changing your own behavior is not easy. Many of us have tried to lose weight, develop exercise routines or stop a bad habit. As we know, it is hard work and often involves repeated successes and failures. Learning to manage tics is also hard work, and for this reason, CBIT has used a number of strategies to help the patient stay motivated. During CBIT, the therapist and patient write down all of the ways in which the tics bother or inconvenience the patient. Each week the patient and therapist review the list and note any changes in the inconveniences. As the patient develops more control over the tics, he or she begins to report fewer and fewer problems caused by tics, and this progress can motivate future efforts.

Can a reward program help with CBIT?

Another strategy, used more with children than adults, is a reward program. In the CBIT reward program, children earn points for attending a session, working hard in session on activities directed by the therapist, and points can also be earned for performing between-session homework assignments. As the child earns more points, he or she becomes eligible for small rewards such as gift cards or computer time. It is important to clarify that these procedures are not used to reward the reduction of tics, rather to reward efforts to use tic management strategies[53-56].

Does CBIT actually work?

Strong evidence supports the effectiveness of CBIT as a treatment for both children and adults with TS. This evidence comes from over 40 years of research on HRT, a primary part of CBIT, and from large, well-controlled research studies on CBIT itself. The research has been conducted on both children and adults.

In one of the best studies on CBIT in children, John Piacentini and colleagues compared CBIT to supportive therapy in 126 children and adolescents with tics. Following eight sessions of therapy, children in the CBIT group had significantly less severe tics than those who received supportive therapy. This benefit was maintained up to six months after treatment ended. Overall, Piacentini found that 52 percent of children going through CBIT were much improved after treatment, and if children got better, they generally stayed better six months later. Sabine Wilhelm and colleagues did another study on adults with tics, and the results were very similar.

Not only does CBIT effectively reduce tics, but there is some evidence that children who successfully complete CBIT will also show less disruptive behavior and anxiety six months after completing the therapy. Furthermore, evidence suggests that CBIT may reduce tics about as effectively as atypical antipsychotics, with the additional benefit of causing no side effects. Overall, data suggest that CBIT is effective. This has led mental health professionals in Europe, Canada and the United States to recommend that when available and desired by patients, CBIT should be a first-line treatment for tics[53-56].

What are other behavioral treatments for tics?

CBIT/HRT has a strong body of evidence supporting its use as a treatment of tics. However, other behavior therapies have been developed and studied. Relaxation training has been tried as a treatment for tics but does not seem to be effective by itself. Early behavior therapists tried things like punishing tics or rewarding patients for not having tics. Neither of these treatments were particularly effective and are not recommended.

There are also other behavioral interventions that appear promising. Based on a treatment performed with obsessive-compulsive disorder, Cara Verdellen and colleagues started using exposure and response prevention (ERP) to treat tics. In ERP, children are encouraged to hold back all of their tics even if experiencing the urges to tic. Over time the patients are encouraged to hold back for longer and longer periods of time. In this therapy, in many cases, they may observe the urges fading away faster and faster. In one study, Verdellen and colleagues showed that ERP was as effective as CBIT but required more therapy time. Another treatment, developed by Canadian psychologist Kieron O'Connor, focused much more on how patients with tics think about and prepare for movement. O'Connor's treatment taught patients to prepare for action in a different way and to recognize and reduce physiological processes that come before and often trigger tics. In preliminary research, this cognitive-psychophysiological treatment has shown promise[53-56].

How do you find a CBIT therapist?

CBIT therapists are not always easy to find, and unfortunately, it is not as easy as looking one up in your local phone directory. The best places to find well trained CBIT therapists are as follows.

1. **Seek therapists who have completed the Tourette Association's Behavior Therapy Institute (BTI).** A few years ago, the TAA developed the BTI to provide formal training to therapists seeking to learn CBIT. Therapists who complete the BTI go through a rigorous training experience led by the developers of CBIT. During this training, they read about CBIT and the CBIT treatment manual. They attend a two-day workshop that involves learning significant details about CBIT and performing a day of practical training where they role play CBIT with mock patients. This practical training is led by the trainers, and during the

training, the therapist learning CBIT is given significant feedback about his or her performance. After the two-day workshop, the therapist-in-training has three follow-up consultations with CBIT trainers. As the therapist works through CBIT with one of his or her actual cases, the CBIT trainer gives guidance, support and suggestions to the trainee. At the end of the three consultations, the therapist is put on a TAA list of providers trained in CBIT. We recommend contacting the TAA or visiting the TAA website to find trained providers in your state and city.

2. **Contact your regional TAA Center of Excellence.** The TAA operates a Tourette Syndrome Center of Excellence program. Any program receiving the Center of Excellence designation, usually offers CBIT. Contacting your local Center of Excellence will provide you with a high quality CBIT referral.

3. **Perform a broad search on the internet for therapists trained in treating TS.** We suggest caution using this approach. As many therapists claim to be able to treat TS, most are not trained in CBIT. If you seek a CBIT therapist through these means, do not be afraid to question the therapist about what they know. Ask them what form of treatment they utilize. If they do not say CBIT, HRT or ERP, or are not familiar with those treatments, we suggest continuing to look for another therapist.

?✦ Secret #3: CBIT is a behavioral therapy that really works to manage tics.

Take Home Points:

- CBIT therapy has been shown to reduce tics in many patients.

- Although for many years behavioral therapy was thought to be ineffective for the treatment of TS, it has now become a mainstream approach.

- Psychoeducation, relaxation and motivation strategies are all important to consider when implementing a behavioral treatment for tic.

- Reward the use of tic reducing strategies, and do not reward the total number of suppressed tics.

- Medications are not always indicated for the treatment of TS.

- Know how to access CBIT and other behavioral therapies. Look for therapists who have completed training.

- CBIT therapists do not have to be counselors or psychologists and frequently are occupational therapists or other advanced care providers.

- Relaxation therapy and exposure response prevention are other approaches to the behavioral treatment of tics. However, there is much less data to support their use in TS.

* * *

CHAPTER 4:

Know When and How to Best Utilize a Social Worker or Counseling Psychologist

"If it's free, it's advice; if you pay for it, it's counseling; if you can use either one, it's a miracle."

— Jack Adams

A FTER THE INITIAL DIAGNOSIS OF TS, the individual receiving the diagnosis as well as his or her family are inevitably left with questions, concerns and fears. What now? Having a name and explanation for puzzling movements, vocalizations and behaviors may not be an answer to more pressing concerns, and it will not likely diminish fears. What can be done to manage symptoms at home? Will the tics get better? Will they become worse? Will my child have friends? Will he or she be able to fulfill academic requirements, graduate high school or go to college? What does this diagnosis mean long term, and to whom can I turn for help?

What is a counseling professional?

Many physicians make a recommendation to follow up with a counseling professional. Counseling professionals include licensed professional counselors, psychologists and social workers who are trained in understanding human behavior, human learning and theories underpinning personal challenges. These professionals offer expertise and use a client's strengths to form interventions aimed at meeting the needs of the client and client family.

When should a counseling professional be engaged in Tourette cases?

When to engage one of these professionals depends on the needs of the family. How is the individual with TS coping? What obstacles are preventing the individual from living the life he or she wants? How are parents, siblings, grandparents and other family members coping? Are there school and friendship issues? If the individual with TS is diagnosed as an adult, how is TS impacting their job, career track, intimate relationships, hobbies and overall well-being? The severity of maladjustment will determine the urgency with which an individual or family seeks help. Generally speaking, individuals seek counseling/social work intervention when their existing coping strategies are no longer effective. In addition, these individuals may need classroom interventions, behavioral modifications, advocacy, resources and therapies aimed at strengthening parenting and interpersonal skills, fostering self-advocacy and building resiliency. Another compelling reason to engage counseling therapy is for the high rate of caregiver burnout.

What are classroom interventions and modifications?

Successes in the classroom and in personal relationships are important goals of living a happier life with TS. Obsessive-Compulsive Disorder (OCD), Attention Deficit Hyperactivity Disorder (ADHD), learning disabilities and depression are common among the Tourette population.

Research suggests that nearly one half of clinic-referred students with TS also have ADHD and OCD[58]; therefore, it is not unusual for a student with TS to encounter difficulties in a classroom setting. Tasks requiring intense focus and concentration can be challenging. Even reading can require great effort, especially when head tossing and eye blinking tics are present. Vocal tics such as throat clearing, sniffing, humming and barking are all disruptive to the individual and to others in the immediate vicinity. School and work situations as well as relationships can understandably become stressful and uneasy. Most teachers today have heard of TS; nonetheless, it is important that classroom performance expectations are congruent with each student's specific needs. Know your educational rights and ask for them. Many clinical psychologists conduct psycho-educational testing to determine if other co-occurring disorders are present. A social worker and counseling psychologist can help determine what accommodations are appropriate and may be helpful for your child. In addition, he or she can attend school meetings and provide emotional and moral support.

My oldest child *(Lydia Breer, mother)* was diagnosed with TS in 1999 when he was five years old. By the time he reached third grade, he was struggling academically. After several frustrating months, an Individualized Education Plan (IEP) was written for him. Adherence to the IEP was my responsibility. I became my son's advocate by educating and working with his teachers and administrators on his behalf. This work was tedious and time consuming. I was exhausted and not very successful because I was too close to the situation to be effective. I eventually enlisted the help of an advocate because of countless unproductive and frustrating meetings with teachers and administrators.

What kind of advocacy is helpful in Tourette?

A professional such as a social worker or counseling psychologist can act on your behalf as an advocate. A few goals of an advocate are 1) educate your audience, 2) voice your concerns and 3) mediate conflicts to reach an agreeable solution with all interested parties. A social worker or counseling psychologist with experience in writing IEPs or one who has some familiarity with advocacy in an education setting is helpful but not necessary. An advocate compassionately communicates "we are all in this together." A team approach reduces resistance to the helping process and encourages collaboration.

Understanding and living with TS from the perspective of siblings, parents and other family members presents its own set of challenges. The unpredictable nature of TS and the waxing and waning of tics is confusing to everyone. Even outside the nuclear family, parents of children with TS can be criticized for bad or poor parenting. This disapproval extends to neighbors, strangers and anyone with whom the family comes in contact. Unsolicited advice, negative comments and dirty looks wear down and demoralize parents and siblings. Here again, the advocate/educator role of a counseling psychologist or social worker is effective in creating a more understanding environment. I will never forget my first family therapy session (Lydia Breer) with a counseling psychologist who asked us to use one word to describe our family. My daughter chose "mad." From her perspective, our family was in a constant state of intense negative emotions. Our counseling psychologist wisely used each of our "one words" to help us understand the "madness" unique to our family. She advocated on my son's behalf. Similarly, I loaned my mother a book explaining TS and its co-occurring disorders. I wanted her to have a firm grasp of the facts regarding TS so she could be supportive of my family and of me. After reading it, she never again uttered a critical word about my parenting. Advocacy is effective in relationships with spouses, friends, co-workers and neighbors. Choose your setting and opportunity and for public discussion. Inviting a helping professional to come speak can be very helpful. Often, support groups form as others want to share their experiences and experience reinforcement. Support groups are an invaluable resource for feeling less isolated and increasing coping skills.

On a larger scale, social workers in particular have training in advocating for legislation and developing social policies aimed at providing needed resources and raising awareness for the TS population. Planning programs that respond to unmet and emerging needs is a central goal of most TS advocacy efforts. Conduct an internet search for a TS non-profit or advocacy group in your city so you, too, can join in their efforts.

What is self-advocacy?

Self-advocacy is perhaps the most important skill to hone. Why? An individual with TS cannot be invisible. Tics don't work that way. There will be times when explaining the vocal and motor tics is necessary. An understanding of your tics and other aspects of your TS diagnosis will help you shape how it is managed. Determining what you need in various situations and settings can help reduce anxiety and stress. A social worker or counseling psychologist can help you learn effective communication skills so that asking for what you need and want is natural and brings about desired results.

What resources are available to Tourette families?

Social workers and counseling psychologists are invaluable resources and provide important connections to services. These professionals network with other helping professionals to assist clients toward their goals and engage in ongoing professional education that is both current and relevant. Continuing education opportunities put them in direct contact with other social workers, psychology and medical professionals such as occupational therapists, nutritionists, homeopathic or holistic practitioners, educators and therapists of various disciplines. Referrals for new and innovative therapies; support groups; camps for children, adults and families; seminars and in-service meetings for parents and teachers; opportunities for social events, fundraising and raising awareness are ways these professionals share their knowledge and connections. In this role, social workers and counseling psychologists act as consultants.

What is an example of a Tourette camp?

One example of a Tourette camp is a Georgia-based program for children ages eight to 17 (http://camptwitchandshout.org.) This week-long camp provides TS patients with opportunities to achieve success, build leadership skills and engage in activities like swimming, a high/low ropes course, boating, a climbing wall, arts, crafts and group activities all with the goal to promote social skills. The camp staff consists of special education teachers and college students studying special education, psychology and social work, and there are also social workers, licensed professional counselors and highly trained nurses and doctors present.

Can support groups be therapeutic?

My oldest son's TS diagnosis *(Lydia Breer)* was just the beginning of a quest to find answers and solutions to challenges and most importantly to find other families and professionals who "got it." I called a local TS organization and spoke with a mom who was parenting a child with TS. She was a medical professional as was her husband. Their connections to the medical community allowed them to provide me with names and phone numbers of other medical professionals so that I could begin addressing my son's tics with medication and later with other approaches. From there, I started my own parent support group and formed two others within my state. These parent support groups offered hope and common ground. We shared information about medications and doctors, nutrition and supplements, exercise, sleep hygiene suggestions and strategies for dealing with teachers and homework. These groups functioned without professional leadership. The disbanding of support groups is natural as children grow, mature and gain the necessary skills to function independently. In addition, parents or others who shepherd those with TS gain skills and confidence to provide support that is independent of the group.

For an individual diagnosed with TS, working on effective interpersonal skills including communication and building confidence are two goals or reasons for joining a therapeutic support group. Therapeutic support groups are different from other support groups in several ways. Therapeutic support groups are led by social workers, counseling psychologists and others trained in mental health. These groups are closed, meaning there are a specific number of members who meet for a fixed period of weeks or months. The goal of this type of group is to understand behavior and promote change. Group members receive feedback that is constructive and delivered in a way that is nonthreatening and conveys both understanding and empathy. Another benefit of being a member of a therapeutic support group is the built-in expectation of pushing through difficult barriers that inhibit change. In a therapeutic safe environment, the individual has the chance to practice new behaviors with the ultimate goal of self-advocacy. A social worker or counseling psychologist who is trained in leading therapeutic groups can keep the momentum going and can provide structure.

Is counseling important in Tourette?

Therapy and counseling are essentially collaborations between the therapist and a client toward shared goals. There are many reasons for seeking the help of a therapist: learn new interpersonal skills and enhance existing ones, heal past wounds, handle disappointments and/or set-backs, gain insight, promote self-determination, build resiliency, change personal goals, adjust to life changes, increase self-regard, enhance a sense of internal control and others. It is important, but not essential, to choose a therapist who has specialized training in the evaluation and treatment of individuals with co-occurring disorders such as TS, OCD, anxiety, depression and ADHD. In any event, it is very important that the client share how he or she experiences TS.

Social workers and counseling psychologists work in a variety of settings such as:

1) Hospitals and clinics, including outpatient clinics and residential facilities

2) Schools and universities

3) Community mental health clinics

4) Dialysis centers

5) Corporations (employee assistance programs)

6) Government agencies

7) Non-profit organizations

8) Home health agencies, such as hospice

9) Private practice

If you work in one of these settings, a mental health professional is an added benefit to you as an employee. Mental health professionals use theories or ideas to provide a framework from which to work through an issue or set of issues. Theories help shape and inform diagnoses. From here, mental health professionals use treatment practices to address the presenting problem. These tools help individuals navigate life stressors and challenges and also utilize personal and environmental factors that help buffer or soften the impact of these stressors and provide resiliency for overcoming adversity.

Can therapists employ behavior strategies?

Behavior therapies can help parents and individuals learn behavior-changing strategies for handling situations that induce stress or anxiety like school or other group settings. Psychotherapy allows individuals to talk about their feelings, deal with set-backs and disappointments explore negative thinking patterns and find ways to effectively manage lives. Parent skills training gives parents an opportunity to work on ways to understand and guide their child's behavior. Likewise, social skills training helps children and adolescents learn and practice new ways of interacting with peers and adults. Some examples include taking turns, understanding personal space, modulation of voice and pacing in conversations, being mindful of the needs of the listener by not dominating conversations, asking questions and using active listening skills. Family therapy provides a non-threatening setting for coping with sibling and parent conflicts and helps strengthen family bonds.

Research shows that strong family bonds are a protective factor in coping with stress[59].

Should self-care be a top priority in Tourette?

When was the last time you flew on a commercial airline? Did you pay attention to the flight attendant spiel? You know the one. Place the oxygen mask on yourself *before* helping others. As a caregiver for someone with TS or if you have TS yourself, it may seem counterintuitive to set self-care as a top priority; however, as the saying goes: "You can't pour from an empty cup" (source unknown).

Just as an athlete trains and fuels his or her body for an endurance sport, caregivers and individuals with TS can and should schedule time, energy and resources, including financial, to meet their emotional, physical and spiritual needs. You would not expect above average or even average job performance from an employee who shows up for work with two hours of sleep and worrisome family issues. Why would you impose these expectations on yourself? Self-care is really self-preservation; it is a necessity. It is a commitment you make to yourself. Here are a few self-care ideas to get you started. You will likely have a few of your own.

1) Outsource. This could include housecleaning, yard work, tutoring your child or carpooling. If money is short, consider tapping into your social or religious network (synagogue, temple, church or small group, Boy Scouts or Girl Scouts, 4-H, Junior Achievement, Rotary, Civitan and Lions Clubs). High school students often want volunteer hours.

2) Date night anyone? Time with your spouse or loved one recharges your connection. If funds are short, consider starting or joining a babysitting co-op.

3) Train your babysitter to be "awesome" so your child looks forward to his or her visit for those times when you just want to recharge doing _____. (You fill in the blank.)

4) Be with people who "get it" and "get" you and your family.

5) Exercise. Yoga, anyone?

6) Eat healthy foods.

7) Drink more water, especially if you are fatigued.

8) Honor your passions: take up something new and fun or indulge your hobby.

9) Journal. Getting it on paper might mean it doesn't roll around in your head, especially at 2 a.m.

10) Meditate or listen to music that expands your soul.

11) Say NO to what does not serve you or bring you joy.

12) Say YES to what does bring you joy.

13) Consider respite care. The Easterseals website (www.easter-seals. com) is a resource. Respite care allows families with children with significant challenges time away to recharge and bond knowing their impacted child is cared for and safe.

Can a social worker or counselor help a Tourette patient and family lead a happier life?

You know your child and yourself best. Nurture passions, innate abilities and gifts. Place your child and yourself in the path of helpers – others who share your goals. Evaluate these helpers thoroughly for the best possible outcome. A TS diagnosis does not define a person. Living a happier life with Tourette syndrome is possible with support from others. Guided by a non-anxious presence; an understanding of the presenting problem; an empathic response and expertise; and help from a social worker, counseling psychologist, licensed professional counselor or other mental health professional can lead to a path of healing, learning and wholeness.

Secret #4: Social workers and counseling psychologists should be employed early and often in Tourette syndrome.

Take Home Points:

- Counseling professionals can be very helpful in TS cases. Licensed clinical social workers and counseling psychologists are both very useful adjuncts to any therapy.

- Using counseling services earlier in the course of TS is preferred to avoid adoption of suboptimal compensatory strategies that can impact later social reintegration.

- Self-care is important for the person with TS and for the family member.

- There are Tourette camps that can be very useful for a subset of children and young adults.

- Counseling professionals can sometimes be certified to deliver TS therapies such as CBIT.

- Learn how to become an advocate for yourself and your child.

- Know where to access resources important for long term management of TS.

- Social workers can help TS patients achieve a happier life.

* * *

CHAPTER 5:

Know When to Pull the Trigger on Medications

"Next to importance in having a good aim is to recognize when to pull the trigger."
— David Letterman

TICS ARE FREQUENTLY DIVERSE IN appearance, complexity and severity. Some individuals have simple eye blinking or head jerking tics, and in many cases these may be tolerable. Others may have extreme or violent movements affecting multiple muscle groups, and these may interfere with daily functioning. Mild tics may not require medication. When tics require a more aggressive approach, medical, behavioral and occasionally surgical options may be considered.

Each person with tics is different, even if another member of the same family also has them. Medication benefits and side effects are highly variable person to person, and a medication response cannot be predicted based upon another person's experience. Most members of society have become accustomed to consulting online reviews to guide travel, purchases and major life decisions. This strategy can be flawed when applied to medical decision-making. The distinct genetics, metabolism and symptoms make each tic patient unique. We recommend that tic patients and caregivers learn a few basic principles and work with an experienced healthcare provider on an individualized plan.

What factor should impact the decision to start medication treatment for Tourette?

Tics by themselves may not be problematic in many cases. However, sometimes tics interfere with daily life or the ability to function in a work or school setting. We recommend as a first step to assess whether the burden of the tics merits the potential risks and benefits of a pharmacological approach to treatment.

- **Physical pain** - Some tics can be bothersome and associated with pain. Typical examples include head snapping or whiplash tics (backward head jerking). These tics can result in muscle soreness, and in rare cases, could even damage the spinal cord. Forceful stretching of muscles or rapid jerking of limbs can also result in muscle and joint pains.

- **Academic or Work Interference** - Tics can affect concentration. If, for example, your tic necessitated that you move your eyes to the side every few seconds, that would be very distracting when reading. Similarly, if your teacher is reviewing important material and you are nodding, tapping and rolling your wrists, you may not be appropriately engaged. It is also possible that in the act of suppressing tics it becomes difficult to focus on a task. Tic suppression is in many cases cognitively distracting. Adults with tics report that job interviews can be daunting. The stress of trying to make a good first impression can result in paradoxical worsening of the tics. Tics may make it hard to function in an office setting and in jobs with direct face-to-face or telephone interaction.

- **Family strain** - Family members with a limited understanding of tics may not tolerate frequent vocal tics or intrusive physical tics. There are cases reported where multiple family members suffer from tics, yet surprisingly, even having a family history of tics does not always equate to the understanding and acceptance of the disorder.

- **Peer relations and social disability** - Tics may in many cases be understood and tolerated by friends and family. Sometimes, however, interpersonal relationships can be negatively affected by the presence of tics. Innocent questioning or requests to "please stop doing that" can produce a sense of rejection and engender feelings of alienation. Peers may react negatively to a constant sniffing or grunting tic especially when it may be distracting, as may occur during a written examination. In more extreme cases, bullying can occur and result in both psychological and physical trauma. People unfamiliar with tics tend to expect that they can be voluntarily controlled. The presence of tics may lead to false assumptions about intellect or personality. Restaurants, airplanes and theaters are closed spaces where peer relations and social interaction can turn negative. If tics interfere with the normal integration into society or the workplace, the risks and benefits of pharmacological intervention may be weighed.

- **Personal distress** - Individuals with tics may have negative self-esteem, which can impact general quality of life. An example would be a person with tics who avoids talking or making friends[60].

Sometimes taking an "inventory" of areas affected by tics, considering all aspects of life, results in the realization that tics are not disturbing function, in which case medication may not be needed. Other times, there may be focal areas that can be addressed with counseling or conservative measures. When these areas cumulatively are impacted enough by tics to detract from good quality of life, however, it may be time to think about treatment. It is critical to remember to focus on the person living with the tics and his or her determination of what is bothersome, rather than introduce medication only on the basis of parental/spousal assumption that tics are disruptive. After considering the above analysis and finding that treatment is needed, there are some basic steps to take to progress on the right path.

How important is finding a good neurologist or psychiatrist to prescribe medications?

A common dilemma when searching for a strategy for medical management of tics is not knowing what kind of doctor to see. The answer depends on both personal factors and regional variations. The majority of individuals with TS experience more than "just tics." In fact, based on one study of 3,500 individuals up to 88 percent have at least one comorbidity, which might include ADHD, OCD, anxiety, depression and others[61]. The types of symptoms impacting a person may make a particular type of doctor more equipped to manage the majority of the symptoms. If severe anxiety is exacerbating the tics and is the major source of distress, or if behavioral difficulties predominate, a psychiatrist may be helpful to manage those comorbidities. However, there are both neurologists and psychiatrists who have good familiarity with tics and their comorbidities as well as experience in treating tics and TS as well as accompanying symptoms. In some cities, a neurologist may be comfortable managing the tics and comorbidities, and in others, a psychiatrist may be the most experienced. It is generally a good idea to start with a primary care doctor and ask who in the area most commonly manages tics or has been a therapeutic ally in terms of working together. Sometimes insurance/payer influences a provider choice. Resources like the Tourette Association of America can be very helpful to identify established experts in tic and TS. Some centers have the capability to provide multiple disciplines of care that collaborate. When this option is available, it is preferred.

What is the start low and go slow rule?

It is easy to escalate doses quickly in TS. However, the goal of therapy is always to control the tics with the lowest effective dose. The side effect risk is often dose-related, meaning that the higher you are on a dose, the greater the chance for encountering intolerance or adverse events. For this reason, it is best to start on low doses and carefully and slowly escalate over time until benefit is attained. If dose-limiting side effects occur, meaning side effects that prevent tolerating any escalation, reducing the dose and changing or adding other therapy may be considered. Going too fast may actually inhibit the ability to fully tolerate a medicine that may work well.

How much time should I give Tourette medicines to work?

By far one of the greatest hindrances to treatment success in TS is an inadequate therapeutic trial. In this case, that means giving up too soon. Tics by definition "wax and wane" over time. That means that if you do nothing, they will fluctuate. Even if you took nothing but sugar candy every day for your TS, you could still have some days of extreme flare ups and some days of relative improvement. If you tried a new pill and the next day had a natural increase in symptoms, you could easily be tempted to blame the pill. If you tried a new pill and had a great few days, you might falsely give the pill credit. Except for the situation of side effects, one should really give a new TS medicine *at least* a few weeks to assess impact. It is also important to remember there is usually a "right" dose required to find that benefit. This trial process takes patience and should include gradual increases over time until the safe, tolerable and effective dose is discovered.

What are realistic goals from drug therapy?

Medication is unlikely to resolve every tic but is likely to reduce the frequency and severity enough to diminish the detriment to function. As a rule, medication should also improve quality of life while improving symptoms.

Once started, are medications for Tourette required forever?

Especially for young people, tics may not be present continuously over a lifetime. In fact, tics often get better or go away by late adolescence or early adulthood[62, 63]. Of course later in life this does not always occur, and tics can get better or worse or change. Once medication therapy is successful and a person is able to enjoy the things important in their life, he or she might wonder if medicine is still necessary. Since some people may "grow out of" tics, it may be that down the road the same medication is not needed. Each person is unique, but one might consider at least six months of being reasonably stable before thinking of weaning off medication. In extremely disabling tic cases, some might find it appropriate to wait a few years before very gently and gradually reducing medications. Of course remaining on medication long term is an option for many patients.

What about the non-tic features?

Comorbidities typically accompany tics. At times, these can be more important than the tics themselves. If these aspects of well-being are ignored, it is unlikely that tics will be maximally controlled. Other medications like antidepressants may be required in select cases.

What about the impact of environmental factors on tics?

No one lives in a vacuum. There are always environmental factors that may help, hurt, nurture or aggravate the situation. It is important to optimize the impact of medications by looking at modifiable life factors that may influence the tics. If tics are better when you play the guitar, capitalize on it. If tics flare up suddenly, think about what stressors may be occurring even when starting or adjusting medication. Is family divorce or another acute stressor occurring? Maybe counseling to help process a life transition would also help the tics. Many individuals with tics find that transitions, in general, may be stressful. This doesn't mean you have to hide from change or eat the same cereal for breakfast every day, but you should key in on fluctuations in tic severity, life factors and social transitions. Time (several weeks) is appropriate before responding with an immediate modification to medication dose or class of medication.

What are the basics on the common Tourette medications?

There are very few drugs currently FDA approved specifically for the indication of tic or TS. At the time of this publication, for adults and children with TS, only haloperidol is approved from ages three and up for TS, and pimozide is approved for severe TS syndrome in ages 12 and up. These drugs have a high risk of side effects and are rarely considered the first line of defense in combatting tics. Additionally, for pediatric patients six to 18 aripiprazole has been approved for TS. Given the limitations in approved options and possible side effects, as elaborated here, current treatment often relies on "off-label" uses of medications. Off-label medications may have a rationale underpinning their use, and if there is emerging evidence from recent clinical trials, that should be monitored by you and your doctor.

What are some recent articles that review medication therapy for Tourette?

Pringsheim, T., Doja, A., Gorman, D., McKinlay, D., Day, L., Billinghurst, L., et al., Canadian guidelines for the evidence-based treatment of tic disorders: pharmacotherapy. Canadian Journal of Psychiatry/ La Revue Canadienne de Psychiatrie. 2012 Mar; 57(3):133-43. PubMed PMID: 22397999[64].

Waldon, K., Hill, J., Termine, C., Balottin, U., Cavanna, A.E., Trials of pharmacological interventions for Tourette syndrome: a systematic review. Behavioural Neurology 2013; 26(4):265-73. PubMed PMID: 22713420[65].

Roessner, V., Plessen, K.J., Rothenberger, A., Ludolph, A.G., Rizzo, R., Skov, L., et al., European clinical guidelines for Tourette syndrome and other tic disorders. Part II: pharmacological treatment. European Child & Adolescent Psychiatry 2011 Apr; 20(4):173-96. PubMed PMID: 21445724. Pubmed Central PMCID: 3065650[66].

Malaty, I. A., and Akbar, U., Updates in medical and surgical therapies for Tourette syndrome. Curr Neurol Neurosci Rep 2014 Jul; 14(7): 458[60].

What are alpha-2 agonists, and can they help in Tourette?

Alpha-2 agonists are medications frequently employed for mild tics, therefore commonly a starting point for treatment of TS. A desirable aspect of this class of medication is the potential to improve ADHD as well as tics. Common side effects include somnolence, low blood pressure and dizziness. Sometimes these medications are helpful, but in many cases stronger pills are needed. This class of medications may also be helpful for anger outbursts.

Can clonidine help with tics and ADHD?

The evidence for clonidine, an alpha-2 agonist used in TS, has been conflicting, but it remains one of the most commonly used medications for tics[60, 64, 67]. Clonidine may also help to supplement ADHD medication and can address impulsivity, which can occur in TS[68]. Clonidine is available in pill form, including extended release, and also in a patch (Catapres). The patch may be useful when swallowing pills is a problem. Doses for oral clonidine usually start at 0.05-0.1mg, and benefit is typically seen at 0.1-0.4mg/day[23, 69]. The maximum dose of clonidine pills is 0.6mg/day. The transdermal (patch) form of clonidine was studied at the 1-2mg daily dose. Possible side effects of clonidine include tiredness, low blood pressure, reduced heart rate, syncope (passing out), dizziness, dry mouth and possible skin reaction (patch). If a decision is made to stop clonidine, it should be weaned gradually instead of stopped suddenly to avoid a rebound increase in tics, blood pressure and increases in anxiety.

Is guanfacine useful in Tourette?

Guanfacine is an alpha-2 agonist and available in short-acting and long-acting forms (Intuniv, Tenex). Similar to clonidine, guanfacine has mixed results in clinical trials but has long been used as an initial drug for TS. Guanfacine has a solid safety profile and has been shown to suppress tics[64, 70-73]. It may also help control irritability and anger outbursts. Tolerability of guanfacine has a similar side effect profile to clonidine and has been associated with sleepiness. However, guanfacine may be less sedating than clonidine, though this effect has not been directly studied. Doses of guanfacine are typically initiated at 0.5-1mg daily, and benefit is observed in most cases at 1-4mg daily. Dosing may be administered once or twice daily[23, 69].

What are neuroleptics (a.k.a. "antipsychotics") and can they be helpful in Tourette?

One hypothesis is that TS results from an overactive dopamine system. Though dopamine is not the only chemical abnormality underpinning TS, strategies that block it have provided a useful treatment. Using dopamine blockers (neuroleptics) was one of the greatest treatment breakthroughs in severe TS[74, 75]. The improvements provided by these drugs offered proof that TS had a biological basis and was not a "psychological" or stress induced disease.

Tic suppression may occur to varying degrees with different antipsychotic agents, but the side effects may be substantial and increase with increasing doses. These medicines are frequently associated with a risk of sedation, weight gain, elevated cholesterol, elevated blood sugar (and diabetes) and temperature regulation issues. Cardiovascular concerns can include low blood pressure, a heart rhythm change called a prolonged QT interval and other abnormal heart rhythms. Hormonal changes could include elevated prolactin (with the exception aripiprazole) which may induce galactorrhea or gynecomastia (milk from breast tissue or abnormal accumulation of breast tissue in males) or amenorrhea (disrupted menstruation). Depression may be a possible side effect. There is risk of akathisia (restlessness) and "extrapyramidal reactions" including tremor, acute dystonic reaction (involuntary muscle activation that can cause twisting postures; not tics) and tardive dyskinesia (other types of involuntary movements that are not tics and could even continue if the medicine is stopped). Tardive dyskinesia, though rare in TS[76, 77], can occur. Neuroleptic malignant syndrome is another rare complication involving increased temperature, blood pressure and muscle stiffness. These issues can be serious or even life-threatening. Some neuroleptics carry an increased risk of liver impairment, low blood counts or increased risk of seizures. Despite the potential for side effects, these medications have a terrific potential to reduce tics, and many TS patients benefit significantly without major side effects. The risks can be minimized by using the lowest dose required to control symptoms.

Typical Neuroleptics
Should I use haloperidol?
Haloperidol was one of the first neuroleptics used for TS. It was FDA approved for both children and adults with TS. Haloperidol has demonstrated benefit consistently in many trials when compared to placebo or to multiple other medications (pimozide, clonidine, fluphenazine, and others); however, the risk of sedation, fatigue and extrapyramidal reactions (Parkinson-like symptoms) was limiting for its use. Although potentially useful for tic benefit, haloperidol carries a very high risk of side effects. For this reason, haloperidol is not considered a first-line TS medication therapy. Doses of haloperidol start at 0.25-0.5mg daily with the typical benefit in the 0.75-5mg daily range (once daily or divided into two doses), but up to 20mg/day doses have been reported[23, 69].

Should I use pimozide for my tics?
Pimozide was the second FDA approved TS medication, and it has similar benefits and side effects to haloperidol. It has shown benefit in multiple trials (compared to placebo, risperidone or haloperidol), and the data supporting its use is similar to haloperidol and to other therapies. Starting doses are 0.5-1mg, and a common range for tic benefit is

2-4mg with a range up to 10mg [23, 69]. Pimozide can cause a prolonged QT interval (heart rhythm issue), so an EKG can be used to screen and monitor. Monitoring is important given the risk of sudden cardiac death[23]. Additionally, a blood test for CTY2D6 status is recommended to confirm whether a person is a fast or slow metabolizer.

Should I take fluphenazine for my tics?
Fluphenazine is another typical dopamine receptor blocker. It may be better tolerated than haloperidol and may provide moderate to marked tic improvement[23, 78]. The starting dose for fluphenazine is 0.5-1mg, with the benefit typically reported at 2-5mg daily[23]. Sleepiness is the most common side effect. Prolonged QT is also a risk (requires EKG monitoring), and fluphenazine should not be given to anyone with narrow-angle glaucoma.

What is an atypical neuroleptic drug?
Atypical neuroleptic drugs tend to have a less potent blockade of D2-type brain dopamine receptors (but work on other receptors). These drugs may in many cases have similar benefits with less adverse effects.

Should I take risperidone for my tics?
Risperidone is an atypical antipsychotic that has been the most studied for use in TS. In trials, risperidone has demonstrated a benefit equal to traditional neuroleptics. Risperidone has also been used for irritability due to autism spectrum disorder. The side effect profile includes a prolonged QT interval (requires EKG monitoring), somnolence and weight gain. Gynecomastia has received a lot of media attention; however, it is not exclusive to risperidone. Doses usually begin at 0.25-0.5mg, and a target dose is typically 2-4mg daily[23, 79].

Should I use quetiapine for my tics?
Quetiapine has been reported to provide improvement in several small studies; however, many were not blinded studies. Sedation and weight gain have been reported as limiting on quetiapine. The dose ranges reported for it are 50-300mg[23, 80, 81].

Should I use olanzapine for my tics?

Olanzapine has been shown to reduce tics in studies including both adults and children. In one six-week study, a 4kg (8.8lb) weight gain was reported. The dose range begins at 2.5mg, and there is a 5-10mg target daily dose[23, 64]. Olanzapine carries a high risk for metabolic disorder and elevated lipids and glucose levels.

Should I use aripiprazole for my tics?

Aripiprazole has been collecting positive evidence supporting a potential short and long term benefit in TS. Tic reduction has been demonstrated in studies that did not mask treatment groups[82] or that studied patients already taking the medicine (82 percent reported significant benefit)[83]. These types of studies, however, can be biased by participant expectation and recall. One 10-week randomized, controlled trial in pediatric patients revealed an improvement in tic scores and a good tolerability with only a mean 1.6kg (3.5 lb) weight gain[84]. A study conducted across multiple Chinese centers showed tic reduction that was equivalent to the established drug tiapride[85].

Should I use ziprasidone for my tics?

Ziprasidone has shown benefit compared to placebo in a small study of 28 patients. The dose range was 5-40mg, and the mean dose was 28.2mg. Currently, the lowest available dose is 20mg. There is a risk of QT prolongation, and EKG monitoring should be employed. Studies are needed to establish the efficacy of ziprasidone in TS[86].

Instead of a dopamine blocker, can I use a dopamine depleter?

Tetrabenazine reduces the packaging of dopamine into vesicles and decreases the amount of dopamine released in the brain. Tetrabenazine accomplishes this endpoint by inhibiting the human vesicular mono-amine transporter type 2 (VMAT2) enzyme. Tetrabenazine has been shown to reduce tics in small studies[23, 87-89]. Better studies are needed; however, expert experience does suggest a potential benefit. Doses start at 12.5mg daily and may range from 50-150mg daily[90]. Some TS patients metabolize tetrabenazine more effectively and tolerate higher doses, whereas others (poor CYP2D6 metabolizers) may be prone to side effects at low dosing. A blood test can reveal which type of metabolizer you are, and this option may be considered if doses must be increased above 50mg/day. The side effects of tetrabenazine can include depression or even suicidality (black box warning), tiredness, low blood pressure, upset stomach and a Parkinson's disease-like state. Weight gain is present but is typically less than with neuroleptics[91]. Tetrabenzine requires monitoring for depression and suicidality especially immediately after initiation of therapy.

Other agents used to treat tic
Should I use topiramate?
Topiramate is an anticonvulsant (seizure medicine) that has been shown to have the potential to reduce tics. It works on sodium channels in the brain and also has an impact on GABA and glutamate neurotransmitter pathways[23]. Topiramate can be helpful when a person with tics also suffers from frequent headaches or seizures, as it is also used for both migraine prevention and seizure control. It is very different from other tic medications. Topiramate tends to suppress appetite rather than increase it like many other TS medications. At least 14 trials have shown similar benefit of using topiramate as compared to other dopamine blocking medicines (e.g. haloperidol, tiapride)[64, 92]. The doses used for tics were variable ranging from 1-9mg/kg/day for children and 50-200mg/day in adults. One study reported the average dose of topiramate was 118mg/day[93]. A recent meta-analysis reported that the quality of evidence for topiramate was insufficient to support the indication for tic suppression, though many experts still use this medication[92]. Topiramate has been reported to cause tingling in the fingers or toes, loss of appetite, weight loss, tiredness, cloudy thinking and word-finding trouble. It may increase the risks of kidney stones and glaucoma. It is therefore important to stay hydrated when taking this medication. Finally, topiramate may cause glaucoma; therefore acute eye pain may require immediately stopping this drug.

Medicines that work on GABA (an inhibitory neurotransmitter/ chemical)

Should I take a benzodiazepine to suppress tics?

Benzodiazepines have been used for a variety of conditions including seizures, sleep disorders, and anxiety. They may also help to reduce tics. Benzodiazepines as a class of medications can be especially helpful if there is a component of anxiety present along with the TS. Clonazepam has revealed evidence supporting tic reduction in small unblinded studies[94-96]. Doses of clonazepam start at 0.25-0.5mg and typically range from 0.5-4mg daily, divided into 1-3 doses/day[23]. Sleepiness or cognitive clouding could be side effects of benzodiazepines. Other side effects include low blood pressure, balance issues/falling and paradoxical reactions meaning agitation instead of the typical tranquilizing effect. This class of medicine may have a mild risk of being habit forming (addictive) in susceptible individuals. If medicine is only taken as prescribed, benzodiazepines in the setting of TS are rarely addictive.

Should I take baclofen for my tics?

Baclofen is not commonly utilized for treatment of tics; however, it does work on the GABA-B receptor and is therefore a reasonable therapy. Baclofen has only been studied in an unblinded fashion, and it has shown a decrease in tics in children treated with about 30mg daily[97]. In practice, that dose is difficult to tolerate without significant sedation. A smaller study of 10 children, examining higher doses did not show statistically significant tic reduction; however, overall improvement on baclofen was reported[23, 98]. The side effects of baclofen include tiredness, constipation, nausea and a risk for withdrawal seizures or psychosis (rare) especially with sudden stopping of the drug. Doses start at 5-10mg two to three times daily and may be escalated to 10-60mg total daily [23, 64, 98].

Should I get injected with botulinum toxin for my tics?

In some cases, the injection of botulinum toxin into specific muscles can lead to a short term relief of motor tics (e.g. about 10-12 weeks) [99-102]. Botulinum toxin inhibits acetylcholine release at the point where the nerve talks to the muscle. This inhibition leads to a reduction in the force of a muscle contraction. There have been unblinded studies and one randomized controlled trial to support this therapy. Botulinum toxin is most likely to be effective for treatment of focal tics causing distress such as painful neck tics. The relaxation of muscles involved may reduce pain, decrease the force of a tic or reduce the urge for that particular tic[100]. However, it should be appreciated that tics cannot always be stopped by simply relaxing the muscle and that with this approach, there is a danger that other tics can become more prominent following injection. Vocal cord injections have been used for severe vocal tics. This approach can occasionally be useful but can also result in softening of speech. There is no antidote to botulinum toxin, so if side effects occur one has to wait until the effect wears off. This can be weeks to months. Risks of botulinum toxin include weakness, bruising, infection, droopy eyelids (blinking injections), swallowing troubles and other issues depending which muscles have been injected and where the toxin may have spread. Though the package information warns of spread of the toxin and even death, the procedure when performed by an expert is quite safe.

What other medications can I try for tics?

Some other classes of medication have been explored for TS. Increasing dopaminergic function by using **dopamine agonists** has shown some tic reduction in early small studies (ropinirole in 15 kids)[103]. However, other studies of dopamine agonists have shown serious risks (pergolide, withdrawn from market for causing heart valve disease) or lack of any tic benefit (pramipexole)[104-106]. **Nicotine** is another approach that stimulates nicotinic acetylcholine receptors. Prior unblinded studies (meaning people knew when they were getting nicotine) revealed that adding nicotine to a neuroleptic might enhance its benefit; however, blinded study (subjects are not told whether they are getting nicotine or placebo) of the nicotine patch demonstrated that it did not significantly reduce tics [107-109]. There are known health risks from the use of nicotine. Other agents that have been tried for TS have included **clozapine** (risk of agranulocytosis), **metoclopramide** (risk of tardive dyskinesia) and **antidepressants**. These all have only small amounts of evidence supporting their use; however, antidepressants can reduce stress and anxiety, and this may indirectly improve motor and vocal tics.

What are some future directions for medication therapy for tics?

A recent search of clinicaltrials.gov reveals the following ongoing or recently completed pharmacologic trials for TS:

- **Two new vesicular monoamine type 2 inhibitors**: These drugs reduce dopamine at nerve terminals. They are tetrabenazine-like drugs, and part of the molecular structure of the drugs is swapped in an effort to enhance tolerability and hopefully improve tic management. NBI-98854 (valbenazine) is currently in Phase 2 clinical trials in TS adults and children. SD-809 (deutetrabenazine) has completed a Phase 1 safety trial in 12 to 18 year olds, but results are currently unavailable on clinicaltrials.gov.

- Once-daily aripiprazole (Abilify) has completed a Phase 3 trial in children and adolescents (7 to 18). Seventy-five of 110 subjects enrolled and completed the trial. They took doses of 5-20mg and were randomized to a treatment group or to a placebo. Publicly available results demonstrate successful tic reduction in YGTSS total tic scores at eight weeks by 13 points in the lower dose group, 18 points in the higher dose group and by only seven points in the placebo group. Some of the side effects reported were nausea, vomiting, somnolence, fatigue, restlessness, increased appetite, headache or other issues. There were no serious adverse events.

- Ecopipam has a novel mechanism of action and selectively blocks the D1/D5 type dopamine receptors. It is hoped that this will interrupt a different component of the circuits involved in TS, and the design of the drug aims at the circuits thought to be involved in faulty excitation. In an open-label eight-week study of 18 adults,

15 completed the trial. YGTSS total tic scores, motor and vocal tics and impairment were reduced with no serious adverse events and no impact on weight gain. Sedation, fatigue, insomnia and somnolence were the most common side effects[110]. A Phase 2 trial in seven to 17 year olds is ongoing.

- Researchers are now paying attention to neurotransmitters other than dopamine, including GABA (an inhibitory neurotransmitter) and glutamate (an excitatory neurotransmitter). Newer drugs may target these chemical systems.

- One recently completed study examined the anticonvulsant (seizure medicine) CPP-109 (vigabatrin) in adults with TS. Vigabatrin utilizes the GABA pathway. In epilepsy, this medication has a black box warning for permanent vision loss.

- There has been interest in drugs affecting glutamate, an excitatory neurotransmitter. Studies have examined both glutamate increasing (D-serine) and glutamate antagonizing/decreasing drugs (riluzole) as compared to placebo. Both types of medicine did not outperform placebo.

- SNC-102 (acamprosate calcium sustained release tablet) has completed a trial in adults with TS. Results are not yet publicly available.

- Abobotulinum toxin (Dysport) vocal cord injection is currently being studied for treatment of vocal tics in TS adults. This drug would relax the vocal cords, potentially decreasing the force generated for vocal tics and possibly modifying the urge to tic.

What are the limitations in current drug studies for Tourette?

The studies that we rely on for guiding tic management often do not offer a complete answer to the symptoms of the syndrome. We are lacking long-term data for many of the drugs used in tic management. The data we do have may utilize doses that don't align with clinical practice. Outcome measures vary between studies, and this impacts our ability to make direct comparisons between available alternatives. Study attrition is also a concern. This is when people drop out of studies, and the benefit is judged from the small group remaining in the cohort. We have come a long way in the last few decades in TS drugs. Ongoing trials of several new tic drugs give us optimism that the future may be even brighter with regard to management options.

❧ Secret #5: Be patient with medication therapy trials for Tourette syndrome since symptoms often wax and wane.

Take Home Points:

- Medications are not always appropriate for treating tics and other symptoms of TS.

- Failure of education and behavioral therapies along with impairment in quality of life is often enough to precipitate using TS medications.

- Potential factors that may influence the use of medications include physical pain, academic or work interference, family strain, problems with peer relationships, social disability and personal distress.

- Start medications at low doses and titrate up slowly to avoid side effects.

- TS symptoms wax and wane, therefore you should wait a month or longer to decide if a particular drug or dose provides meaningful benefits.

- A reasonably safe class of medications often employed to suppress tics are alpha-2 agonists (guanfacine and clonidine).

- A more aggressive approach to suppress tics is to use dopamine blocking agents. Often atypical antipsychotics (e.g. risperidone) are used to reduce side effects, rather than jumping to typical agents (e.g. haloperidol).

- Dopamine blockers used in TS can be associated with sleepiness and weight gain but rarely are associated with tardive dyskinesia (abnormal extra movements in the face and potentially body).

- Dopamine depleters like tetrabenazine seem to be safer than dopamine blockers in some aspects but also can be associated with severe depression and suicidality (requires monitoring).

- Injecting botulinum toxin for focal tics may be a reasonable therapy.

* * *

CHAPTER 6:

Should I Make My Brain Electric?

"What is a soul? It's like electricity – we don't really know what it is, but it's a force that can light a room."

— Ray Charles

How did DBS become a chronic therapy for tremor and other neurological diseases?

ALIM BENABID, AN ACCOMPLISHED DOCTOR, was not known beyond his specialized field. He was a professor of neurosurgery at the Joseph Fourier University in Grenoble, France from 1978 to 2007. His routine duties included treating people debilitated by the symptoms of Parkinson's disease by placing small lesions into deep regions within their brains. One day, Benabid had a "what if" moment that would forever alter the treatment of Parkinson's disease and tremor. More importantly, it would radically and positively impact the lives of many sufferers.

On the operating room table was an elderly man who was afflicted by pain and tremors. Benabid utilized a technique referred to as intraoperative mapping, and as a routine he gathered a detailed physiological brain map. Benabid would obsessively check and double check his map to confirm localization of the "sweet spot." He was aware from his thousands of hours of intraoperative experience that the sweet spot was the precise location within the brain that if tickled would result in relief of Parkinson's symptoms. He also knew that if he missed the spot there would be no relief, and in some cases it could precipitate severe side effects.

Benabid passed a large test probe several centimeters below the brain's surface. Initially, the results were as he predicted; the tremor worsened when he stimulated through the probe with a series of very slow pulses. In contrast, it improved when he stimulated with faster pulses. What happened next was the real breakthrough. Instead of burning a hole in the brain, Benabid decided to change course. It would be hard to not overstate the significance of this moment because of the tens of thousands of Parkinson's disease and tremor patients whose lives would be forever transformed by that decision. Instead of heating the tip of the test probe and placing a tiny lesion deep inside the brain, he withdrew it and placed what would later be referred to as a DBS lead[111-117].

Prior to Benabid's use of a chronically-implanted DBS lead to treat the symptoms of Parkinson's disease, conventional treatment was to make a brain lesion to "disrupt the disruption" in a rogue brain circuit that was stuck in a state of abnormal oscillation.

One of the amazing observations about the human brain is that its normal functions seem to be dictated by rhythmic oscillations that continuously repeat over and over, much like a popular song on the radio. The oscillations change and modulate, and they act to control various human behaviors. If an oscillation "goes bad," it can result in a disabling tremor or alternatively in many of the other symptoms of Parkinson's disease.

That day in the operating room, Alim Benabid decided to remove the lesion probe he had used hundreds of times before and replace it with a wire that had four metal contacts at the tip. This wire, later referred to as a deep brain stimulation (DBS) lead, was connected to an external battery source. Benabid and his neurology colleagues could program the device using a small old-fashioned box with several small buttons and archaic looking switches. As simple as the system appeared, it turned out to be very powerful, allowing Benabid to individualize the settings to a possible 12,000+ combinations. Unlike lesion therapy, this new approach provided Benabid and his team a tailored or personalized medical solution to many of the disabling symptoms of Parkinson's disease and of tremor[111-118].

How does DBS work?

Since DBS likely works in many ways (electrical, chemical, excitation and/or jamming inhibition), we now believe that the electrical current sets off a complex symphony of coordinated information transfers between many brain elements and regions. This complex information transfer ultimately leads to improvement in symptoms. Since so many regions are involved in this coordinated response, we refer to this as a neural network[118]. Phil Starr, a neurosurgeon at the University of California, San Francisco, has shown that there is a complex relationship between the cells stimulated deep in the brain and the cerebral cortex in Parkinson's disease patients[119]. When the DBS device is turned on, the cells in the two regions become coherent and fire in a new synchrony. Ayse Gunduz and colleagues at the University of Florida have shown in a similar experiment that Tourette DBS results in reverse changes in the brain than observed in Parkinson's disease. We have not yet unlocked the mechanism of action of DBS, though we do now understand many of the biological changes that may occur in response to the electricity[120].

Is an interdisciplinary team approach important in DBS for Tourette?

DBS drove a worldwide movement toward better interdisciplinary care for the Parkinson's disease patient. Prior to DBS, most care was delivered in isolation by physicians, nurses, nurse practitioners or physician assistants. The complexities of screening a DBS candidate would, in contrast to typical care, require a multidisciplinary approach. A neurologist, neurosurgeon, psychologist, radiologist and psychiatrist would all participate in a comprehensive evaluation. Over time, physical therapists, occupational therapists, speech therapists and social workers would, as a result of this process, transform into important members of this team. Together the team would make critical surgical decisions, and individually each team member would become an expert in his or her field.

Ultimately so many people participated in the care of a single DBS patient that the process gradually shifted from multidisciplinary to interdisciplinary. Interdisciplinary care is the highest level of a patient-centric experience, and it has been utilized for decades by cancer centers and rehabilitation hospitals. Interdisciplinary care involves specialists sitting together and discussing an individual patient, which stands in contrast to consultative or multidisciplinary care, in which practitioners communicate by sending notes or letters to each other. For Parkinson's disease, the birth of the interdisciplinary DBS evaluation greatly enhanced the level of care and has forged dramatic improvements in patient and family satisfaction. DBS, a surgical not medical procedure, would transform and improve the care for all Parkinson's disease patients, even those not receiving an operation[118, 121-124]. Tourette, like other indications for DBS, should also utilize interdisciplinary care.

What do they actually do during DBS surgery?

The DBS procedure is a marvel of modern medicine. It requires only a dime-sized hole in the skull. The operation is performed in virtual reality on a computer screen and within minutes can be translated into a human patient. The surgeon can navigate around blood vessels and refine a region of interest to reach within a few millimeters of an intended target. A few millimeters may be small on a ruler, but it is very large in brain space. A few millimeters of brain space can be compared to the distance between Florida and California.

The surgical team can thread several microelectrodes into a Parkinson's disease patient's brain to record and to develop a three dimensional map. This map includes both the desired target location and also the position of surrounding brain structures. There are many brain targets that can be chosen for a patient. The choice of target is usually tailored during a detailed discussion, which involves the patient and his or her DBS team. The complete map is a critical part of the DBS procedure itself because if the final DBS lead is misplaced by even a few millimeters, it can be the difference between dramatic success and miserable failure. Failure could mean a lack of benefit but could also mean that a patient is left with permanent stroke-like symptoms. Using microelectrodes to define a region is more important in Parkinson's disease than in TS. In TS excellent neuroimaging may be enough for some of the targets (e.g. CM thalamus); however, imaging alone may not be enough for other targets (e.g. GPi).

Once the final location for the DBS lead has been determined, it can be locked into place by a capping device. A connector wire can be attached and tunneled underneath the skin. In one final step, a battery, referred to as a neurostimulator, can be placed under the collarbone. The neurostimulator is like a cardiac pacemaker[118, 121-124].

How is the DBS device tuned once implanted?

Once placed, a neurologist or advanced practice provider can cycle through thousands of possible DBS programming parameters in order to optimize the settings for a patient. Optimization of the settings usually takes a few weeks to a few months and can lead to exquisite control of the many disabling symptoms of Parkinson's disease such as tremor, stiffness, slowness and in some cases even walking[118, 121-124].

How will Tourette DBS, which is not FDA approved, advance and improve in the future?

One remarkable fact about DBS therapy is that the hardware has changed very little since Benabid's experiment. The brain lead, the connector wires and the battery technologies have only been slightly improved. The FDA currently has approved two DBS devices for Parkinson's disease patients and one for epilepsy, and it is well known that better technologies are languishing as they snake their way through the trenches of a difficult FDA approval process. Tourette DBS is not approved by the FDA. The techniques for delivering currents and for securing the electrodes remain fundamentally unchanged. Despite the lack of a new DBS technology, penetration of the device into communities all over the world has been explosive, with nearly 125,000 Parkinson's and movement disorders patients having been transformed into bionic existences.

So what will it take to move the TS DBS field forward? A critical first step will be to develop an understanding of the needs of the TS patients. Patients and families currently seek treatment to address the symptoms that are not adequately covered by medications and behavioral therapy. Second, the therapy will need to be safe, and clinical trials will need to be sufficiently robust and demonstrate benefit greater than the placebo effect (e.g. improvement greater than would be predicted by chance). Third, the therapy must be cost effective and incrementally better than all existing therapies. Any hope of moving the technology and ultimately the field forward will need to address these three major hurdles.

What improvements are we likely to see in the DBS device itself?

There have been important and recent research advances in DBS device development. First, there are many new DBS lead designs. Most of the new designs will enable the electrical current to be administered to more specific regions of the brain, thereby enhancing benefits and reducing side effects. Second, the type of electrical current we now utilize is referred to as a voltage-driven, non-steered system. In this voltage-driven paradigm, there can be shifts over time in the actual size and shape of the electrical field that is delivered to the brain tissue. Also, current stimulators do not steer current toward desirable regions or away from undesirable ones. Newer stimulators will use a constant current device that will smooth tissue delivery and improve the effectiveness of the therapy, and leads will be segmented and allow steering. A third issue that has emerged is battery life. Clinicians and patients have a critical need for longer lasting, and in some cases, rechargeable batteries. Better battery lives will mean fewer replacement surgeries and less of a chance for battery failure and return of symptoms. These new approaches and products have already begun to appear and are working their way through the FDA approval process.

Patients have also begun to demand sleeker and smaller devices as a box protruding from the chest area is unattractive and undesirable. It would also be preferable to most patients to eliminate the connector wire that attaches the lead in the head to the box in the chest, In TS this is particularly important as the connector can be damaged by thrusts of the neck during motor tics. Finally, it would be ideal to be able to program the device from a remote location. Imagine the day when a doctor can see you by video and tune your device without the need to change out of your pajamas or leave your house. All of these advances are coming soon[125-127].

Could DBS be tailored for specific symptoms?

Another encouraging development is the ability to tailor or personalize a therapy for an individual patient. With all the advancements in DBS, it may be possible to hone in on specific bothersome symptoms. For example, one brain target may be best for motor tics and another for vocal tics or OCD. Patients would choose the target based on their needs. Also, we are no longer limited to one or even two DBS brain leads. The ability to place multiple DBS leads into a single patient over time as his or her disease evolves and new symptoms emerge is quickly becoming a reality.

Since tics are paroxysmal, could we develop a smart DBS device?

The newest Holy Grail in DBS will be the development of a biomarker. The National Institutes of Health defines a biomarker as "a characteristic that is objectively measured and evaluated as an indicator of normal biologic processes, pathogenic processes, or pharmacologic responses to a therapeutic intervention." In layman's terms, a biomarker is an indicator that one has or does not have a disease (i.e. a blood test that may reveal the diagnosis of Parkinson's disease). When it comes to the electric brain, scientists have raised the possibility of an electrical biomarker. The general idea is that disease activity could be monitored by an electrical signal that is being naturally emitted by specific brain regions. So instead of using the biomarker to diagnose the disease, doctors would use the abnormal electrical patterns to direct treatment, in this case, electrical treatment of TS.

It has now become recently possible to record the brain after DBS and capture the signals in real time. Previously, the brain could only be recorded during the actual operating room procedure. The type of signal that can now be collected is called a local field potential or LFP. LFPs are special measurements of the brain's native electrical current and also its inherent oscillatory properties. In TS, research has revealed an important LFP called the alpha band. This band changes when patients tic. Understanding electrical biomarkers will allow the development of smarter devices. The hope is that new devices will sense a particular abnormality, like an alpha band, and automatically respond. The result is called an on-demand paradigm. In on-demand circuits, electrical abnormalities can be addressed by applying current to the brain. The idea of on-demand systems is to solve brain problems as they emerge and before the development of a particular clinical issue or symptom. Thus the era of personalized medicine has arrived[128].

What do we know about the outcomes for TS DBS?

TS DBS has not achieved FDA approval and very few cases have been performed worldwide. The relative number of TS cases resulting in severe enough disability to merit surgical intervention is low; therefore, it is unlikely a single center will accumulate a large enough number of cases and outcomes to significantly influence the field. The Tourette Association of America recently funded an international multi-center

SHOULD I MAKE MY BRAIN ELECTRIC?

effort to register cases and share outcomes data. Additionally, the group has revised recommendations for TS DBS patient selection. Currently, less than 200 cases are being followed with the most common targets being the CM thalamic region, the GPi (motor and also limbic territories) and the ventral striatum/ventral capsule accumbens region. Most of the collective experience has been in CM and GPi, and there seems to be 30 percent plus improvement in motor and vocal tics, with less consistent benefits in other behavioral features. The range of improvement has been wide with a subset of patients doing very well, while others experience a suboptimal outcome and may request explant (removal of the leads and devices). The most important message is that DBS is not a cure, and though it is a powerful symptomatic treatment, suppression of tics may not always lead to an improved quality of life[129].

I am interested in DBS. What's next?

A review and updated recommendations[126] was recently published in the journal Movement Disorders. The most important element for success in TS DBS is undergoing a complete multidisciplinary screening inclusive of neurology, psychiatry, neurosurgery, and in many cases physical, occupational, speech and swallow therapy. We also now routinely utilize counselors or social workers to educate patients and families and to align expectations which are often and understandably inflated. Good candidates must have a DSM V diagnosis of TS and have exhausted medical and behavioral therapies. The motor and/or vocal tics must be disabling. Other psychiatric comorbidities such as anxiety disorder, depression or bipolar disorder must be optimally treated and stable prior to an operation. Past or present suicidality must be addressed by the screening team and could be an exclusionary criterion. Once all members of a DBS screening team have evaluated the potential candidate, a group discussion format should be used to vet candidacy and to decide surgical approach, targets and follow up. DBS is not the right therapy for every TS patient, and you should not be disappointed if a multidisciplinary team recommends against proceeding with a surgical intervention[126].

Who pays for TS DBS in the United States?

TS DBS is not FDA approved, therefore if the expense is not fully covered by research grants or other funding, it may not be reimbursed by insurance. Each insurance carrier is different, and recently we uncovered a disturbing trend of pre-authorization for DBS implantation but failure to pay the bill. These types of bait and switch tactics have proven frustrating for patients and families in need of DBS surgery for medication and behaviorally refractory tics[130].

?❧ Secret #6: Utilize an experienced multidisciplinary DBS screening team if you are considering making your brain electric.

Take Home Points:

- DBS surgery is not FDA approved for TS and is not appropriate for all TS patients.

- Careful multi-disciplinary screening should be employed in all cases, and the recent recommendations from the Tourette Association of America are a reasonable guideline.

- TS patients with malignant tics and those with head snapping tics that have a risk of cervical spine injury may be potential candidates.

- The most appropriate brain targets, surgical procedures, programming and management remain unknown; however, there is an International Deep Brain Stimulation Registry and Database for Gilles de la Tourette Syndrome tracking outcomes in an effort to better guide the field.

- Most TS patients who have DBS have an approximate 30 to 50 percent benefit in motor and/or vocal tics. Much less is known about OCD and other symptoms when DBS is employed in the current preferred brain targets for TS DBS (thalamus and globus pallidus).

- The OCD associated with DBS may not respond as positively as primary OCD disorders implanted in the anterior limb of the internal capsule/nucleus accumbens region.

- The complication rate seems to be higher with TS DBS inclusive of infections, hardware issues and need for device removal (explants).

- Since DBS is not FDA approved, patients and families should be cautious as DBS may be pre-approved by a medical director of an insurance company, but the bill may not be paid (bait and switch). This bait and switch scenario may also apply to battery replacements, and in the future rechargeable devices may be preferred for TS DBS.

Much of this DBS-related chapter was reproduced and updated with permission from the publisher and author Okun, M.S., Parkinson's Treatment: 10 Secrets to a Happier Life. Createspace, 2013.

* * *

CHAPTER 7:

Should I be thinking about transcranial magnetic stimulation (TMS) and other novel techniques?

"Magnetism, as you recall from physics class, is a powerful force that causes certain items to be attracted to refrigerators."

— Dave Barry

How did we get from the electric torpedo fish to electro-convulsive therapy?

DELIVERING EXTERNAL ENERGY INTO THE human body to treat physical ailments is not a novel concept. Scribonius Largus, a physician for Emperor Claudius of ancient Rome, used an electric torpedo ray fish to treat headaches.[131] Dr. Gilles de la Tourette, after whom Tourette Syndrome (TS) was named, developed a "vibrating helmet" to treat various neurological conditions.[132]

What is ECT?

Electroconvulsive therapy (ECT) was developed in 1938 by Ugo Cerletti to treat schizophrenia but has subsequently been used to treat other psychiatric conditions including major depression. ECT is performed by delivering a sufficiently strong electrical current through the scalp and skull such that a short-lasting seizure occurs. Prior to the routine use of anesthesia and muscle relaxants, ECT-provoked seizures resulted in bone fractures and joint dislocations. The currently used ECT procedures in most centers utilize general anesthesia and muscle paralytics to prevent body convulsions. Not long after its initial debut, ECT was used to treat a patient with "florid tics".[133, 134] Since then, only a handful of medical reports have described the use of ECT in chronic tic patients. There are collectively fewer than 10 patients described in the medical literature who have received ECT for tic therapy, and there have been mixed outcomes.[135-138] Although a form of non-invasive brain stimulation, ECT is not a benign treatment option since a controlled seizure occurs as part of the therapy. ECT is currently not a widely recommended therapy in TS unless accompanied by medication resistant depression.

What is transcranial magnetic stimulation (TMS)?

Transcranial magnetic stimulation (TMS) was developed in 1985. Although the name of this technology implies that magnetism is what directly stimulates the brain, what actually happens is the TMS machine uses fluxing magnetic fields to induce a very small electrical current. The ingenuity behind this technology is the TMS device produces magnetic fields that painlessly penetrate the scalp and skull to eventually induce this small electrical current on the surface of the brain. This electrical current can be used to stimulate brain cells.

How does TMS work?

The basic design of TMS involves three main components – a high-voltage power supply, a capacitor and a stimulator coil. The power supply typically charges the capacitor to 1 to 3 kilovolts. Power can then be discharged to create a time-varying magnetic field through the stimulator coil, which is made of tightly wound copper wires. The end result of the system is the creation of a TMS pulse. This TMS pulse induces a small electrical current that stimulates the brain. The electrical current induction is an example of Faraday's law of induction which is a basic physics law about electromagnetism. A quick internet search for Faraday's law will provide examples of this concept.

How has TMS evolved as a research and clinical tool?

The earliest human TMS studies focused on the brain regions that activate the arms and legs. These studies are relatively straightforward to conduct because a single TMS pulse can trigger muscle contractions that can be easily measured. More complicated stimulation protocols have now been developed ranging from paired pulses delivered very closely together, separated only by a few milliseconds, to over 1,000 pulses delivered in a 20 to 30 minute interval. Each of these different stimulation protocols allows scientists to measure different properties of the human brain tissue. Using the single TMS pulse method, one can measure how excitable the brain is – the motor threshold. Measurement of the muscle contraction (motor-evoked potential) after a TMS pulse also allows the quantification of the speed and extent of motor system activation. Another important property that can be measured is the efficiency of the brain's braking system (cortical inhibition). This can be achieved by using different single- and paired-pulse TMS procedures. The final TMS paradigm that will be discussed is repetitive TMS (rTMS), which involves the delivery of multiple TMS pulses ranging from hundreds to more than a thousand pulses per session. Studies in healthy volunteers, mostly adults with few pediatric reports, demonstrate that rTMS can temporarily change the excitability of brain circuits; therefore laying the foundation for investigative trials utilizing rTMS to treat TS patients.

What is the safety and tolerability of TMS? Does it cause seizures?

An important question for researchers has been to address safety and tolerability issues of this technology. Fortunately, most side effects from TMS are mild and short-lasting (headaches, scalp discomfort). Children also tolerate TMS relatively well.[139] There are concerns about negative impact on hearing as each TMS pulse produces a clicking sound. Appropriate earplugs should be worn during TMS sessions, especially if the stimulation intensity is high. There are rare reports of subjects passing out during TMS sessions, but this is not believed to be directly related to TMS.[140] The most serious concern is that research participants have developed seizures that were thought to be provoked by TMS. This is most concerning with rTMS (repetitive TMS) as multiple pulses are delivered per session; therefore, more external energy is imparted into the brain. International TMS researchers have met in response to various safety concerns and published two consensus statements on the use and safety of TMS.[140, 141] Currently, the international TMS community states that single- and paired-pulse TMS studies are relatively safe, even for children as young as two years old. However, these consensus statements do recommend limits on stimulation parameters for certain rTMS protocols. Unfortunately, there is limited medical literature on newer rTMS techniques such as theta burst stimulation (TBS); therefore, consensus is still lacking on appropriate parameters for TBS. So far there is only one published report of TBS-induced seizure, and based on preliminary data, TBS-induced seizures are likely infrequent.[142-144]

Could TMS be used to predict treatment success in Tourette or even as a potential treatment?

Potential clinical applications for TMS fall under two main categories. The first is using TMS to measure physiologic properties to potentially predict treatment outcomes. The rationale here is that each TMS measurement is directly dependent on specific brain chemical (neurotransmitter) systems and that tic-reducing medications can modulate these neurotransmitter systems. Furthermore, cognitive tasks have been shown in TMS experiments to alter the motor system; therefore, it may be possible to use this technology to predict response to Comprehensive Behavioral Intervention for Tics (CBIT). The second category is the use of rTMS to modulate brain circuits to eventually decrease tics.

Could physiological measures predict treatment outcome?

There are several adult and pediatric TMS studies showing that the excitability of the motor system is different in TS patients when compared to age-matched controls.[145-148] These motor system outputs are also measures that have been shown to be regulated by mental manipulations.[149, 150] Therefore, it may be possible to conduct specific baseline TMS measurements to predict CBIT response.

Multiple studies have demonstrated the presence of an abnormal cortical inhibition (braking system) in TS adults and children.[145, 146, 151-154] More importantly, the deficit in cortical inhibition can correlate with higher tic severity.[145, 153] The neurotransmitter GABA system is involved in these TMS measures, and pharmacologic agents that act on the GABA system such as baclofen and clonazepam can be used to treat tics.[98, 155]

Although rTMS is often thought of as a therapeutic intervention, these protocols can actually characterize the brain's innate property to adapt and modify (i.e. neuroplasticity). Various rTMS paradigms have demonstrated that neuroplasticity may be altered in TS patients.[156-160] These measures are highly dependent on a balanced dopamine system, which is the primary target of numerous medications for tic therapy (dopamine receptor agonist/antagonist, dopamine depleter).[161]

Thus many experts have concluded that based on the pharmacology of TMS measures, TS disease mechanism, medication properties and cognitive research, it may be possible to use various TMS measures to predict treatment outcomes from medications and/or CBIT.

Can rTMS be used to reduce tics?

By the early 1990s, emerging research data suggested that rTMS could modulate brain activity and potentially be used as a therapeutic tool. Currently, rTMS has only one FDA cleared indication for treatment, which is for major depression. However, interest in using rTMS to treat TS dates back to the late 1990s.[162] To date, there are only a handful of published rTMS studies treating tics. Before discussing the available data, it is worthwhile to briefly discuss issues regarding rTMS clinical trial design. There is currently no standardized recommendation on how to best deliver rTMS; therefore, significant variabilities exist between studies. Therapeutic rTMS trials require identification of a stimulation target. This target identification has not been consistent in TS trials as earlier studies focused on primary motor and premotor regions. The primary motor region is the area of the brain that when stimulated causes direct muscle activation, while the premotor region is a pre-planning motor area that ultimately contributes to execution of motor movements. More recently, rTMS-TS studies have targeted the supplementary motor area (SMA) as this region has been suggested to be a critical area responsible for tic formation.

The most ideal TS study design is one that is randomized (some patients get active whereas others get sham/placebo stimulation), sham-controlled (placebo stimulation) and double-blinded (neither the patients nor the researchers are aware which randomization the patients received). So far, published studies indicate that all TS patients who participated in rTMS trials have tolerated various study protocols without any serious adverse events. The hope is that future studies will adopt more rigorous methods.

What are the outcomes of low-frequency TMS studies?

Earlier rTMS-TS studies focused on stimulation of the primary motor or premotor regions. These studies mostly used low-frequency 1 Hz rTMS, which is thought to decrease brain excitability. Using this low-frequency rTMS, investigators theorized that tics may subside if activity over the primary motor or premotor regions were reduced by rTMS. The results were mixed. In Alexander Münchau's study[163], adult TS patients received active stimulation to the left primary motor or left premotor region or alternatively had sham stimulation to the left primary motor region. For each randomized condition, each patient received two stimulation sessions over two consecutive days. Twelve patients completed this study, but no statistically significant reduction in tics was detected. Orth et al. published a slightly more complex study using 1 Hz rTMS to target premotor regions.[152, 164] This study design had three different protocols: 1) active stimulation of left premotor followed by right premotor area, 2) active left premotor stimulation followed by sham right premotor area and 3) sham stimulation of left premotor area followed by sham stimulation of the right premotor area. Five adults received two rTMS sessions over two consecutive days and were randomized to the three different protocols. Statistical analysis also failed to reveal a meaningful reduction in tic severity. Chae et al.[165] took a slightly different approach. This group used both 1 Hz rTMS and also a higher-frequency TMS approach (15 Hz rTMS). Higher-frequency rTMS is thought to facilitate brain activity rather than suppress it. Stimulation targets were either the primary motor or the prefrontal cortex. Eight adult participants were randomized to sham, 1 Hz or 15 Hz rTMS and also to primary motor versus prefrontal stimulation. There was no statistically significant change in tic severity based on self-report or videotaped review.

What were the outcomes of TMS when the motor planning area of the brain was targeted?

There were several studies undertaken to target the motor planning region of the brain in TS (the SMA). Most studies used 1 Hz rTMS and a much longer stimulation course (≥ 2 weeks), with only one exception. Two of the six studies included a sham control group. These TMS studies also included significantly more pediatric patients than previous investigations. The stimulation course was two days for one study[166], two weeks for two smaller studies[167, 168], three weeks for one study (20 adults)[169], four weeks for one pediatric study (25 kids)[170] and 12 weeks for another pediatric study (10 kids)[171]. All of the studies without a sham control demonstrated a variable degree of tic reduction. The three-week stimulation study[169] was a two-site, randomized, double-blinded and sham controlled study. This design was ideal for a TMS clinical trial. Of the 20 adults who completed this study, nine received active rTMS while 11 received sham rTMS. Tic severity for the active rTMS group decreased after three weeks of therapy. However, interestingly the sham group also experienced tic reduction, and the final analysis did not reveal a statistically significant difference between the two groups.

What about using theta burst stimulation (TBS) to treat Tourette?

TBS is a newer form of rTMS that has two advantages over 1 Hz rTMS. First, the stimulation duration is much shorter. The protocol used was less than one minute per session whereas 1 Hz rTMS usually takes 20 to 30 minutes per session. The stimulation intensity was lower than what is required for 1 Hz rTMS. Twelve subjects (two adults, 10 kids) completed this study with six in the active TBS group and six in the sham TBS group. Each patient received a randomized stimulation condition for four sessions per day for two consecutive days. Investigators also used functional brain MRI to determine each patient's specific sweet spot for SMA stimulation. This imaging information was used along with a neuronavigation system to target the TMS coil to each individual's SMA region. Prior to this study, SMA targeting has all been performed based on rough scalp measurements. The results revealed that there was no difference in tic reduction between the two groups. However, the motor system activity was observed to be significantly different between the two groups when assessed by functional brain MRI following active TBS treatments.

What about using transcranial electrical stimulation (tES) for treatment of Tourette?

There are currently two other forms of transcranial electrical stimulation other than electroconvulsive therapy (ECT). These techniques are called transcranial direct current stimulation and transcranial alternating current stimulation (tACS). TDCS was introduced in the 1990s and has more published research data. The technology uses a weak direct electrical current, usually in the range of 1-2 milliamps in an effort to modulate brain activity. The application of tDCS requires a power source that uses ordinary home-used batteries to deliver a weak electrical current through two or more electrode surface(s). One electrode is set as either the negative or positive contact while the other electrode(s) are designated as the opposite polarity. The electrical current, by convention, travels from the negative contact toward the positive contact(s). The stimulation duration usually ranges from approximately 10 to 20 minutes per session. The dosing of tDCS depends on current density and stimulation duration. The initial description of tDCS used two surfaces which contacted the scalp. The electrical stimulation delivered through this setup was less focused compared to more recently developed high-density (HD) tDCS. HD tDCS uses one central electrode with multiple surrounding electrodes to deliver the current. This setup provides a more specific stimulation of a targeted brain region.

tACS is a different form of transcranial electrical stimulation that delivers an alternating electrical current. Since the current alternates between positive and negative polarities, there are no fixed positive and negative contacts over the scalp. The main goal of tACS has been to modulate brain oscillatory activities.

Is tDCS safe?

tDCS has been used more than tACS. Based on available data, tDCS is relatively safe but not without potential concerns. The procedure is tolerated relatively well with subjects complaining of mild side effects such as scalp itchiness/redness, headaches and tiredness. One case of seizure has been reported possibly relating to tDCS.[172] It was a four-year-old child who experienced a seizure four hours after the third tDCS session. This seizure was preceded by two prior daily tDCS. There were multiple factors that could possibly have explained why this child had a seizure, so it is possible that this event was completely unrelated to tDCS administration.

Should I make my own homemade tDCS device?

It is worthwhile to note that the internet has provided an avenue for the public to construct homemade tDCS devices. A word of caution must be raised because non-invasive transcranial electrical stimulation should not be performed outside of a research setting. Although available data suggests that this technology is relatively safe, the scientific community is not aware of long term positive or negative effects. Other factors may also affect the safety profile, such as variations in individual brain anatomy, differences in skull thickness, other medical conditions (e.g. heart disease) and age. Furthermore, ideal and safe stimulation parameters have not been established for TS therapy. We do not recommend you order the parts and make your own tDCS machine.

What are the outcomes from tDCS used to treat Tourette?

To date, there are only two patients (both adults) reported to have received tDCS for experimental therapy.[173] Each subject received five days of active stimulation and five days of sham stimulation separated by two weeks. The electrode (cathode) placement in this study reduced the activity of the left primary motor and premotor regions. Both participants tolerated the stimulation well. Self-reported tics decreased after the active stimulation but not after sham stimulation. Although promising, it is difficult to conclude about tDCS efficacy in tic treatment from a small case series of two patients.

What are the challenges of non-invasive brain stimulation trials and future directions?

There are multiple variables that can potentially explain the mixed results for rTMS-TS studies. Target selection is a critical decision. Based on brain imaging studies, the SMA is considered an important region for tic generation. However, there are also other areas that activate immediately before tic execution. The current approach has focused on suppressing SMA activity in hopes that tics will decrease by targeting this region.

Another investigative approach involves activating the region(s) that are responsible for suppressing tics. This new approach could serve to enhance a patient's abilities to suppress tics. This is analogous to strategies used in other diseases that use rTMS. In these other diseases the aim is to directly activate the injured region to promote recovery.

The techniques for TMS and tDCS may be variable, and we are not sure of the best overall technique. Once the stimulation target(s) are identified, the ideal study design is to individualize the stimulation procedure by utilizing neuronavigation technology. For example, although the SMA can be anatomically defined on structural brain MRI images, functional activation-based localization of the SMA may vary from person to person. It would make sense to target the rTMS stimulation coil to each individual's exact functional SMA area, rather than just using scalp measurements or anatomical structures.

Another challenge is how long the stimulation should be administered to patients. Several published studies have subjects come in daily during the weekdays for several weeks. This is very difficult for most people due to home, school and work demands. In fact, one study reported that this factor was the greatest challenge in recruitment.[169] The stimulation course must be long enough to provide benefit but not too long that it hampers people's lives. This issue could possibly be potentially addressed by combining rTMS with CBIT to promote faster tic reduction. This potential approach is also similar to motor rehabilitation studies that combine rTMS with physical and occupational therapies.

There are multiple confounders or factors that may impact outcome of TS studies. The presence of co-occurring conditions (e.g. ADD/ADHD, OCD), prescription medication(s), prior medication history and duration of symptoms all can affect the interpretation of clinical trials. It is impossible to eliminate all of these confounding factors; therefore, rigorous statistical analyses must be employed, and interpretation must be performed carefully.

TOURETTE SYNDROME: 10 SECRETS TO A HAPPIER LIFE

Adequacy of sham control is important for clinical trials to tease out a potential placebo effect. Depending on the rTMS protocol, sham stimulation may be easier to figure out. For example, for 1 Hz rTMS, the stimulation intensity is often set near or above the motor threshold. This means the stimulation is generally higher, and the subject is more likely to feel twitching of scalp muscles, whereas sham stimulation does not produce any muscle twitching. In the most recently published double-blinded study[169], a relatively low percentage of blinded investigators and subjects were able to correctly identify the stimulation condition. Not surprisingly, research participants (24 percent) were better than investigators (14 percent) at identifying active versus sham rTMS.

What is the promise of brain stimulation for TS?

Brain stimulation is an old concept. However, technological advancement has provided safer and more precise methods. Current non-invasive brain stimulation techniques hold promise in treating TS. Further understanding in structural and functional neuroanatomy, careful study design and optimal stimulation techniques are required to potentially establish non-invasive brain stimulation as a therapeutic option for TS.

❧ Secret #7: Transcranial magnetic and direct current stimulation, though safe, are not ready for prime time as Tourette syndrome therapies.

Take Home Messages:

- TMS is a safe technique that rarely results in side effects and rarely, if ever, is associated with seizures.

- TMS currents can be applied to the brain at low and high frequency to study the circuitry underlying TS.

- TMS may also in the future be used as a tool to predict response to therapy.

- There are very few treatment trials using TS for tics and other TS-related symptoms, and the results have not (to date) been impressive.

- tDCS is another technique that is evolving for clinical and research use. Very few trials have been performed. Both TMS and tDCS may be limited by the small amounts of current applied to the brain and also how deep the current can penetrate.

- Clinical and research targets in the brain such as the SMA and cerebellum may provide important clues to the circuitry under-pinning tics and may also provide information on novel targets and approaches for treatment.

* * *

CHAPTER 8:

What do I need to know about PANDAS?

"It is a colossal task for the immune system to maintain tolerance to self and yet be ready to react to everything in the world around us."

— Bruce Beutler

What is PANDAS?

PANDAS, SHORT FOR PEDIATRIC AUTOIMMUNE Neuropsychiatric Disorder Associated with Streptococcal infection, is a form of obsessive-compulsive disorder (OCD) and tic disorder(s) in children and adolescents that is triggered by streptococcal infection(s). PANDAS is a subset of proposed broader categories known as Pediatric Acute-onset Neuropsychiatric Syndrome (PANS) or Childhood Acute Neuropsychiatric Symptoms (CANS). We primarily focus on PANDAS as it better encompasses tic related disorders. PANDAS was first written about in the mid-1990s, although infectious triggers for tics and abnormal behaviors where originally published in the early 1900s. Children with PANDAS have a sudden and severe onset of OCD or tics, as well as at least two other new neuropsychiatric symptoms, such as anxiety, irritability, aggression, behavioral regression (acting younger than they are), sensory processing abnormalities (sensitivities or hallucinations) and/or sleep disturbances [174].

What causes PANDAS?

PANDAS is thought to be caused by a common infectious bacteria known as Group A Streptococcus (GAS), otherwise known as *Streptococcus pyogenes*. This bacterium routinely causes pharyngitis (also known as strep throat), sinusitis and ear infections. Though these infections can be concerning, most treated children will experience little long term effect, with very few developing secondary reactive arthritis or acute renal inflammation (glomerulonephritis). Rarely patients may develop a more serious complication called rheumatic fever, which is a serious autoimmune condition involving the heart, joints, skin and brain that develops several weeks after the infection.

How is PANDAS different from rheumatic fever?

The neurological presentation of rheumatic fever, Sydenham's chorea (SC), occurs when GAS infections trigger an immune response in the body that leads to production of antibodies that normally target and fight the infection. Instead, these antibodies begin targeting cells in the brain, primarily in a region called the basal ganglia. The basal ganglia is the part of the brain that regulates emotions, basic behaviors and physical movements. When these antibodies pass through the blood-brain barrier, inflammation and interruption of the normal functioning of neurons (cells of the central nervous system) develops. The antibodies involved attack dopamine 2 receptors [175] leading to abnormal movements (chorea), weakness and behavioral disturbances. A similar process is thought to occur in PANDAS, but instead of abnormal movements (chorea), weakness and behavior disturbances, OCD, changes in behavior and abnormal movements (tics) are predominantly seen. It should be noted that while there is some overlap in presentation, SC may present with rheumatic carditis, whereas PANDAS is not associated with heart inflammation.

Who gets PANDAS?

Typically, PANDAS presents in children ages three through puberty. The rate of occurrence dramatically diminishes after 12, but a few cases have been noted in adolescence and rarely in adults. The average age of onset is around 7.3 years old. Similar to non- PANDAS tics and OCD, it occurs more often in boys than girls [176].

How often does PANDAS occur?

The precise prevalence of PANDAS is unknown. It is estimated that there are 500,000 children with OCD in the United States, and approximately 138,000 children with TS [177]. Of these, it is estimated that up to 25 percent of children with OCD and/or tics may meet most of the PANDAS diagnostic criteria. Some children may present with evidence of GAS trigger but have less of a dramatic onset. Some may have a relatively sudden and severe onset but with less definitive evidence of a GAS association. Meeting all criteria is less common; for example, one study found that 11 percent of TS patients had an abrupt onset of tics induced by a streptococcal infection[178].

What is the relationship of the PANDAS symptoms to the infection? Can it be related to a family history of autoimmune conditions?

PANDAS symptoms (e.g., OCD, tics, restricted food intake, etc.) often present during or shortly after the GAS infection. Alternatively, PANS/CANS is associated with infections or causes other than GAS; these might include mycoplasma or viral respiratory infections. Some of these children may have weakened immune systems, thus it is not surprising to observe a positive association between children who have frequent upper respiratory infections and a history of tonsillectomy and/ or adenoidectomy [179]. Research has also found that there is a correlation between those with a maternal family history of autoimmune conditions and those who develop PANDAS [180] or tics [181].

How does PANDAS present?

According to recent diagnostic guidelines, the primary presentation of PANDAS is rapid-onset OCD that is accompanied by one or more additional symptoms, including tics. Differentiating PANDAS from non-immune OCD is the rapidity and severity of onset. Typically, symptoms of classical OCD take weeks to months to fully develop. However, in the case of PANDAS, there is an abrupt onset in which the child will go from being healthy to experiencing severe symptoms over the course of one to two days. These children often do not present with just tics or OCD; rather, they often have many comorbid neuropsychiatric symptoms (Table 1).

Table 1. PANDAS Characteristics	
Male gender	67-72% (N=112)
OCD	86-100% (N=112)
Tics	33-81% (N=112)
ADHD	40-61% (N=112)
Emotional lability	59-84% (N=112)
Psychosis	12% (N=41)
Separation anxiety	29-74% (N=112)
Enuresis (involuntary urination)	12-42% (N=112)
Choreiform movements (very mild chorea like movements)	42-78% (N=112)
Frequent urination	42-78% (N=62)
Handwriting deterioration	29-61% (N=112)

174, 182, 183

What is required to diagnose PANDAS?

There are no definitive laboratory tests to diagnose PANDAS. Diagnosis is based on clinical history and the association of symptoms with streptococcal infection at or around the time of onset. Lab work and imaging procedures are used to rule out other conditions and guide treatment. The diagnostic criteria are:

- Presence of clinically significant obsessions and compulsions and/or tic disorder

- Pre-pubertal onset of symptoms

- Abrupt onset of symptoms and/or relapsing-remitting course

- Temporal association with streptococcal infection

- Association with other neuropsychiatric symptoms

Keep in mind that PANDAS is a diagnosis of exclusion and is not solely contingent upon meeting criteria, meaning other physiological and psychological causes of the patient's symptoms must be ruled out prior to establishing the diagnosis. This means that a child cannot be diagnosed with PANDAS if his or her symptoms are better explained by another disease, disorder or condition. Further, some cases that have similarities in presentation and symptoms to those seen in PANDAS may fall into the broader category of PANS.

When PANDAS is being considered as a diagnosis, establishing a streptococcal or other associated infection is important though not necessary for classification as PANS/CANS. An identified specific trigger aids in treatment decisions, so it is important to obtain this information whenever feasible. However, the period between infection and onset of symptoms can be highly variable, making it difficult at times to establish a relationship between infection and symptoms. Typically, the interval is one to 10 days. The best way to establish a relationship between symptom onset and an infection is by showing that streptococcal bacteria (or other infectious triggers) are present in the child when symptoms begin. This can be done through the use of rapid streptococcal antigen testing in the doctor's office or by throat culture. Testing the blood for streptococcal, mycoplasma, influenza and other viral antibodies (also known as titers) may be helpful; however, this will only tell the clinician if there has been an infection in the past and does not mean that the infection is currently active. Sometimes titers remain elevated for months or for life, as with certain viruses and mycoplasma.

In addition to establishing the presence of an infection, it is important for families to keep a record of when and how the child's symptoms occurred, the severity of the symptoms, when/if the symptoms remit and when/if they reoccur. Other helpful information could be records of medication use (e.g. antibiotics and psychotropic medications) and also include over-the-counter medicines and supplements. Noting the name of an antibiotic, the dose and the duration of treatment is useful. Obtaining pediatric records that document illness and treatment is helpful as well.

What are the immune-based therapies used to treat PANDAS?

Therapies that target the body's immune response are ideally the first line of treatment for PANS/PANDAS. Immune-based therapies include the use of antibiotics, non-steroidal anti-inflammatory drugs (NSAIDS), steroids, intravenous immunoglobulin (IVIG) and plasmapheresis.

Antibiotics work by targeting bacteria and slowing down antibody production, reducing localized and systemic inflammation. Sometimes an extended course of antibiotics is necessary, and providers may follow prophylactic antibiotic guidelines for the treatment of rheumatic fever. Prophylactic antibiotics help to reduce the risk of new infections, thus reducing PANDAS symptom flares [184]. There are some risks with extended use of antibiotics (e.g. macrolides like azithromycin) which may cause prolonged QTc (on EKG), increase the risk of an allergic response, deplete 'good' bacteria in the gut and contribute to antibiotic resistance.

Risks versus benefits should always be considered when contemplating such treatments. Steroids and NSAIDS have been observed to be helpful at times, but more research is needed to examine risks and benefits.

What are treatments for PANDAS cases that do not respond to antibiotics?

Many PANDAS cases may spontaneously remit over time. However, in more severe or persistent cases, more intense treatments may be necessary. Generally these children are more severely ill and have many different neuropsychiatric presentations such as severe OCD, mood disturbances, sleep disturbances and food refusal. Tics may or may not be present and are often not as impairing as the other symptoms.

Options for more intense treatments include plasma exchange or IVIG. IVIG therapy is the process of delivering immunoglobulins, a type of antibody, to the blood via intravenous infusion. These infusions contain helpful antibodies pooled from the plasma of many donors that help in the suppression of the patient's own abnormal antibodies, thus reducing their negative impact. IVIG is sometimes effective in reducing symptoms with some indications of greater response in patients with immune deficiencies. Some initial response should be observed within one month, but it may take several months to see an optimal response to IVIG. Often only one infusion is necessary, but the optimal number of infusions is not known. Plasmapheresis works by filtering the blood to remove plasma, which contains antibodies, reducing the body's autoimmune reactions for a time. This treatment carries a higher risk and should be used only when other options have failed and symptoms remain severe and problematic. There have been studies showing that both plasma exchange or IVIG are helpful for PANDAS or infection-triggered OCD and tics [185, 186], and further research is needed to establish which patients are likely to respond as well as dosing and frequency guidelines for the treatment of PANDAS patients.

Are tonsillectomies and adenoidectomies useful to treat PANDAS?

There have been some studies that support the benefits of tonsillectomies and adenoidectomies in reducing PANDAS flares [187]; however, the evidence is mainly in the form of case reports. There is still much controversy over effectiveness. Tonsillectomies and adenoidectomies are a common treatment for severe and recurring strep infections, but they have no indication in the treatment of PANDAS, except for cases in which the surgical guidelines are met. Examples include demonstrated obstructive sleep apnea or refractory chronic pharyngitis. Murphy, Lewin, Parker-Athill, Storch and Mutch [179] found that many PANDAS patients had a history of tonsillectomy and adenoidectomy prior to the onset of PANDAS, which may indicate that tonsillectomies and adenoidectomies predispose patients to PANDAS. No differences were observed in laboratory markers and symptom severity in youth with PANDAS with and without a surgical history.

Are the typical medications used to treat OCD, ADHD and tics useful to treat PANDAS?

In addition to immune therapies, PANDAS symptoms can be treated similarly to their non-PANDAS counterparts. For example, OCD in a child with PANDAS can be treated with selective serotonin reuptake inhibitors (SSRIs), just as in non-PANDAS OCD. Symptoms of ADHD are sometimes associated with PANDAS and can be treated with stimulants, as would non-PANDAS ADHD. Tics may be treated with medications typically used to treat non-PANDAS tics, such as alpha-2 agonists or antipsychotics. However, it is highly recommended that medications be initiated one at a time and at lower starting doses than would typically be used for other diseases. This reduces the possibility of behavioral activation (agitation, mood lability) which is often seen in children with PANDAS.

What about behavioral therapies to address the symptoms of PANDAS?

In addition to medical therapy, behavioral therapies have been found to be helpful in reducing symptom severity in children with PANDAS. Cognitive behavioral therapy (CBT) helps patients and parents by providing strategies to change behaviors and patterns of thinking and to reduce anxiety. Parents also learn strategies for addressing externalized symptoms such as tantrums and aggression. CBT is a standard treatment for non-PANDAS OCD and has been found to be very effective in reducing symptom severity. Habit reversal training (HRT) is a standard treatment for tics, skin picking and hair pulling (trichotillomania). HRT aims to increase behavioral awareness and replace the impairing behaviors with alternative and more acceptable behaviors.

Occupational therapy (OT) may help address the deterioration of fine motor skills that many children with PANDAS experience. OT has been found useful in addressing areas such as implementing adaptive routines, making environmental modifications, utilizing sensory tools and assistive technologies and teaching stress management techniques [188]. Responses to treatment vary with some patients completely regaining their fine motor skills and others reporting continued symptoms.

My child has PANDAS. Now what?

If you believe that your child has a PANDAS spectrum disorder (i.e. their course of symptoms matches closely with those discussed above), you may be wondering where to turn next. You should begin by consulting with your child's pediatrician or primary care doctor. Further evaluations and referrals to psychiatry, psychology and neurology are likely indicated. The PANDAS network website (www.pandasnetwork. org) is a great resource for finding providers with experience treating PANDAS. The PANDAS Provider Network (www.pandasppn.org) is a good resource for providing initial information to your doctors if they are unfamiliar with the topic.

What does the future hold for PANDAS?

Looking to the future, more research is needed to establish a greater understanding of this condition, particularly regarding its autoimmune nature. Treatment guidelines will need to be established. A multimodal approach that includes research in the areas of psychiatry, neurology, rheumatology, immunology and genetics could lead to a greater understanding of the causes and treatments of PANDAS. As medical research is currently progressing at an unprecedented pace, we are hopeful that future research will yield further insight. For the time being, we hope to see continued expansion of efforts to raise awareness and support for children with PANDAS, including the establishment of guidelines and recommendations to assist the wider medical field in prompt and evidence-based treatments.

❧ Secret #8: PANDAS is uncommon and sometimes confused with Tourette syndrome.

Take Home Points:

- PANDAS is a relatively rare disorder and may be mistaken for TS. Some experts believe that many of the suspected PANDAS cases actually have TS. PANDAS cases seem to have a more abrupt onset of symptoms, present with many other difficulties like anxiety, mood, eating problems and sudden change in school performance when compared to TS.

- PANDAS belongs to a family of disorders called autoimmune syndromes. Autoimmune issues may be triggered by infections that accidentally trigger an immune response against the brain (e.g. the basal ganglia) resulting in potential movement and behavioral abnormalities.

- PANDAS is associated with many of the same behavioral issues seen in TS and is closely associated with OCD.

- The diagnosis of PANDAS requires expertise in the area and a careful history and neurological examination. It is a tricky diagnosis and one of exclusion, meaning the doctor must exclude all other causes including TS before declaring it a PANDAS case. There should be presence of clinically significant obsessions and compulsions and/or tic disorder, a pre-pubertal onset of symptoms, an abrupt onset of symptoms and/or relapsing-remitting course, temporal association with streptococcal infection and an association with other neuropsychiatric symptoms.

- The same behavioral and medical treatments for TS can be applied to many PANDAS cases.

- Treatment with antibiotics, IVIG, anti-inflammatories and steroids have all been suggested, though it is not clear at this time who to treat, when to treat and what agent to use in treating a sufferer. In uncertain cases, empiric antibiotics therapy is not recommended because of the risk for antibiotic-resistant infections.

* * *

CHAPTER 9:

What should I know about marijuana?

"I have [...] come to the realization that it is irresponsible not to provide the best care we can as a medical community, care that could involve marijuana."

— Dr. Sanjay Gupta

IN RECENT YEARS, THERE HAS been an increase in media attention on the subject of medical marijuana for various neurological conditions. Most of the attention has focused on the treatment of seizures and multiple sclerosis (MS), but we are often asked in the clinic setting what is known about medical marijuana for Tourette syndrome (TS) and other movement disorders. Although there is some hope it may be effective for some of the symptoms of TS, the research and research funding has been limited.

What is medical marijuana?

The terms medical marijuana and medical cannabis are often used by the public and by medical professionals interchangeably. Broadly, these terms refer to the use of marijuana or compounds derived from the cannabis plant and compounds that are utilized for the treatment of specific medical symptoms. Technically, the term marijuana refers specifically to the raw form of dried flower buds that are derived from the cannabis plant. Cannabis is a more general term that refers to any part of the actual cannabis plant. The term cannabinoid refers to the chemical compounds contained within the cannabis plant. The cannabis plant contains two major cannabinoid compounds, and both have been extracted for medical use. One is Δ-9-tetrahydrocannabinol (THC). This compound is thought to be the psychoactive component of marijuana. The other is cannabidiol (CBD). This compound is thought to be a non-psychoactive component of the plant. Plants can be purposely bred to contain a higher ratio of a desired cannabinoid compound. Δ-9-THC has been the compound most studied in TS. CBD is the compound most studied for seizures[191, 192].

What are the three main forms of cannabis?

There are three main forms of cannabis[191, 192]:

1) Marijuana (dried buds for vaporizing, smoking, eating)

   a. Plant strains with varying percentages of Δ-9-THC versus CBD

2) Cannabis extracts (oils, pills, oral sprays)

   a. Pure Δ-9-THC

   b. Pure CBD

   c. Combinations of Δ-9-THC and CBD (one pharmaceutical oral spray called Nabiximols/Sativex, one pharmaceutical pill called Cannador)

3) Pharmaceutically synthesized (pills)

   a. Δ-9-THC (two pharmaceutical pills called Dronabinol/Marinol and Nabilone/Cesamet)

How accessible is marijuana, and what is the legal status?

There is a split between the U.S. federal government and many state governments over medical marijuana policy. Under United States federal law, it is illegal to possess, use, buy, sell or cultivate cannabis; however, a growing number of states have recently approved marijuana for medical use. Cannabis is a Schedule I drug under the Federal Controlled Substances Act, meaning it has been defined to have a high potential for abuse and in the federal government's opinion has no acceptable medicinal use. This schedule renders cannabis use illegal for any reason with the exception of FDA and DEA-approved research programs.

The FDA drug standard classification for drugs ranges from Schedule I to Schedule V. FDA classification of marijuana as a Schedule I drug limits the potential for research. There has been a push from scientists and researchers to change the classification of cannabis from Schedule I to Schedule IV or Schedule V to facilitate research. For now, cannabis remains Schedule I, but Nabilone/Cesamet is Schedule II and Dronabinol/Marinol is Schedule III.

Despite the Schedule I classification, in recent years several states have passed laws that allow possession and sale of marijuana for medicinal, and in some cases, recreational use. In these circumstances, the states with medical marijuana laws generally do not prosecute individuals for the possession or sale of marijuana as long as they are in compliance with the state's marijuana regulations. In many states where medical marijuana is available, a doctor may "recommend" the drug, and a patient may obtain a medical card or the equivalent to purchase cannabis or a cannabinoid extract from a licensed dispensary. Pharmaceutical formulations are available by prescription only and are only FDA approved for appetite stimulation in AIDS and for chemotherapy-induced nausea and vomiting.

What is the rationale for marijuana use in Tourette?

It is scientifically reasonable to believe that cannabinoids may be a useful adjunctive therapy in TS. Cannabinoids occur naturally in the body, and cannabinoid receptors are found throughout many brain regions. In the 1990s two types of receptors were identified and described: CB1 and CB2. CB1 receptors are located in high concentrations in regions of the brain thought to be involved in TS (e.g. the basal ganglia). It is believed that marijuana and Δ-9-THC both work on CB1 receptors. CB1 receptors can be bound by cannabinoids that occur naturally in the body; alternatively, these receptors can be bound by drugs or other compounds. When the receptors are bound they are thought to affect neurochemicals and suppress or modulate inappropriate brain signaling[191, 192].

What research supports a possible benefit in TS?

Surveys, anecdotal reports and small uncontrolled case studies have suggested a possible benefit for marijuana in TS patients. There are only two controlled studies of using cannabinoids in TS. Both studies utilized pharmaceutically synthesized Δ-9-THC sold as Dronabinol/Marinol. It is important to realize that although many patients with TS are children, these studies were focused exclusively on adults. The first study was conducted in Germany in 2002 by Kirsten Müller-Vahl and enrolled 12 patients[191, 192]. Each patient was administered a single dose of either a Δ-9-THC pill or a placebo pill. Four weeks later, patients were administered a single dose of the alternate drug (either a Δ-9-THC pill or a placebo pill). TS patients were then rated before the dose and four hours after. Patients rated symptoms of impulse control, obsessive-compulsive behavior, anxiety, depression, ADHD and urge to tic. The study was double-blinded, meaning that neither patients nor doctors were aware of the type of pill taken. Ten patients reported benefit after Δ-9-THC, and three reported benefit after placebo. There was also a significant patient reported reduction in vocal tics, motor tics and obsessive-compulsive behavior. On examiner ratings scales, there was a significant improvement in complex motor tics. The size of the effect was small, and it was not present across all rating scales. No serious adverse events were reported, but mild transient adverse reactions were reported in five patients. Though this study suggested a possible benefit, not enough patients were studied to draw reliable conclusions about either safety or efficacy.

The second study was conducted by the same research team in 2003[191, 192]. Twenty-four patients received either Δ-9-THC or placebo for a six-week trial period. The Δ-9-THC patients received increasing doses every four days until reaching the target dose. Tic severity was rated by the examiner using several rating scales, and the ratings were scored at six visits. Patients also rated tics and premonitory urges. The results showed an improvement in tics at the target dose of Δ-9-THC when rated by the examiner and the patient. Again, the degree of improvement was relatively small, and there was not a significant difference on all of the scales. When further statistical analysis was performed to account for multiple comparisons, the improvements that were seen on some scales no longer reached statistical significance. Eight of the 24 patients participated in the previous study. This repeat participation introduced a selection bias, as patients who had a benefit in the first study may have been more likely to volunteer for another study. Additionally, seven of the 24 patients dropped out of the study and were not included in the results. This introduced attrition bias because people experiencing the least amount of benefit were more likely to drop out. Regarding side effects, one patient dropped out due to anxiety and restlessness, and five patients reported mild symptoms such as tiredness, dry mouth, dizziness and cognitive clouding.

Do any Tourette experts favor the use of marijuana?

Overall, though both of these studies revealed a trend toward benefit, both were too short, too small and had other technical limitations. In 2014, the American Academy of Neurology concluded that based on these studies the data was insufficient to support or to refute the efficacy of Δ-9-THC for reducing tic severity[193]. A Cochrane systematic review of the literature (performed by an independent, non-profit, non-governmental organization) drew the same conclusion[194]. There are, however, many researchers who acknowledge the limitations of current studies but feel strongly that in treatment-resistant patients, cannabis may be tried[192]. Despite disagreement between experts about the appropriateness of cannabis for TS, there is a general consensus that longer research trials with larger numbers of patients will be necessary to establish the long term effectiveness and safety of cannabinoids.

What are the risks and other considerations for cannabis use in Tourette?

In a 2014 review in the New England Journal of Medicine, the director of the National Institute on Drug Abuse carefully described the adverse health effects of marijuana use[195]. Below we outline these effects as well as other considerations[196]:

- Smoking is the most common way people use marijuana, and this can harm the lungs.

- With oral forms, the amount in the bloodstream can be uncertain due to unpredictable breakdown by the liver and accumulation in fat.

- Tolerance can develop, and approximately nine percent of users will become addicted.

- There may be a withdrawal syndrome that can make quitting difficult for some users.

- Use in adolescence and early adulthood can contribute to worsening brain function, decreased connections between brain regions and a decrease in IQ.

- Heavy marijuana use can rarely lead to psychosis and hallucinations.

- Marijuana can reduce cognitive and motor function. The risk of car accident doubles if you have recently smoked marijuana.

- The potency of the THC content in marijuana has increased from three percent to 12 percent in the last several decades making accidental overdoses, especially with food products, much more common.

- The best evidence supporting marijuana use has been shown in glaucoma, nausea, AIDS wasting syndrome, chronic pain, multiple sclerosis and epilepsy.

- Many patients with Tourette syndrome are children. The risks of marijuana and cannabinoids to children are probably much higher than adults but have not been studied.

- There are synthetic cannabinoid compounds being manufactured by pharmaceutical companies as mentioned above, but there are also synthetic cannabis products being sold on the internet and in tobacco specialty shops. These are completely different than pharmaceutical compounds. They are usually marketed as incense not for human consumption and contain chemical compounds sprayed onto an herbal base material. They are sold under names such as Spice and K2. These are unpredictable, can have severe neurologic and systemic side effects and should be avoided.

Should I consider using synthetic cannabinoids for my Tourette?

Patients need to be aware that since Woodstock there have been changes in the availability and types of marijuana. The most important thing to be aware of is the burgeoning market for synthetic cannabinoids. A synthetic or manufactured version of marijuana may be similar to THC but different elements of the structure can be altered. There are many formulations including those that can be smoked, eaten (powders) or sold as teas. Perhaps the most well-known synthetic version of marijuana has been sold under the name Spice. Other common product names include Kronic, Northern Lights, K2, Zeus, Puff, Tai High, Aroma, K2, fake weed, Yucatan Fire, Skunk, Moon Rocks and Magic Dragon. Though

Spice and other synthetic cannabinoids may be illegal in many states, manufacturers may skirt state and federal laws by replacing and manipulating chemicals in the synthetic version. Experiences with synthetic versions of marijuana have not always been positive. There has been a recent surge of patients visiting emergency rooms after ingesting synthetic cannabinoids. Rapid heart rates, vomiting, agitation, confusion and hallucinations have all been reported. Poison control centers have also recently reported an uptick in synthetic cannabinoid toxicity. Additionally, there have been withdrawal and addiction symptoms reported with some formulations. Because of the current safety issues most expert practitioners discourage synthetic cannabinoid use for TS, though there may be a brighter horizon in the future as more is learned[196].

Considering the evidence, is it reasonable to think marijuana has a role in treating Tourette?

While there is reason to believe that medical marijuana may be helpful for TS, it has not been rigorously studied. Benefits are not proven, risks are not well understood and legal status remains an issue. This is, however, a potentially promising area in need of further study as specific TS symptoms may in the future be found to benefit from marijuana.

✷ Secret #9: Marijuana may have both risks and benefits when employed to treat Tourette syndrome symptoms.

Take Home Points:

- Medical marijuana and medical cannabis are terms used by the public and medical professionals interchangeably.

- These are compounds derived from the cannabis plant and compounds that are utilized for the treatment of specific medical symptoms.

- Marijuana refers specifically to the raw form of dried flower buds that are derived from the cannabis plant.

- Cannabis is a more general term that refers to any part of the actual cannabis plant.

- Cannabinoid refers to the two major chemical compounds contained within the cannabis plant. Both have been extracted for medical use. One is Δ-9-tetrahydrocannabidol (THC). This compound is thought to be the psychoactive component of marijuana. The other is cannabidiol (CBD). This compound is thought to be a non-psychoactive component of the plant.

- Δ-9-THC has been the compound most studied in TS, whereas CBD is the compound most studied with seizures.

- There is some accumulating evidence that marijuana may be useful in the treatment of at least some of the symptoms of TS (tics and non-motor symptoms). More research is needed to better define for which symptoms and which patients marijuana would be appropriate.

- There are potential dangers to using marijuana, especially damage to the lungs if inhaled as well as an increased risk for car crashes. Risks to the developing brain are not well understood.

- At this time, synthetic marijuana compounds are not recommended due to the high risk of contaminants and reported cases of morbidity and mortality.

- Relaxation of the federal legal classification of marijuana may help researchers study medicinal marijuana for TS and other neurological diseases.

* * *

CHAPTER 10:

What are future directions for Tourette research?

"If you do not change your direction, you may end up where you are heading."
— Lao Tzu

SINCE TOURETTE SYNDROME (TS) WAS recognized in the 1800's, there have been intense, international research efforts aimed at determining the risk factors and causes associated with its development[197]. Studies have focused on deciphering the brain changes underlying the symptoms as well as trying to understand the natural history of these conditions. There continue to be multiple approaches to the development of treatments for individuals with TS and other tic disorders.

What are the recent advances in understanding the development of Tourette?

The discovery of TS has led to a protracted period of speculation as to potential underlying cause(s)[198]. Much of the early speculation lacked scientific evidence to support claims. Tics have been proposed to be caused by evil spirts and immoral behaviors. Recent research has evolved into multiple lines of rational hypothesis-driven investigations primarily aimed at determining genetic, environmental, lifestyle and other factors underlying the etiology of TS.

Family, twin and segregation studies (whether a dominant or recessive trait) have consistently supported hereditary factors as underlying the development of TS. TS has been linked genetically to other tic disorders and associated conditions such as OCD and ADHD[23, 199]. However, linkage and other genetic studies have to date failed to determine the precise mode of transmission, and these studies have also not identified genetic risk loci and associated genes. A recent study identified alterations in the L-histidine decarboxylase gene in a family with TS, though patients should understand this is a very rare gene mutation[23, 199, 200].

More recent research approaches have employed copy number variation studies. This means sections of DNA can be repeated and number of repeats per person can vary. These experiments utilize a technique called microarrays. The microarrays can be used to decipher small structural variations and determine the genetic changes associated with TS. Emerging studies have identified various potential candidate loci and genes, as well as possible links to other neurodevelopmental conditions such as autism spectrum disorders[201]. Similarly, genome wide association studies, which can detect small disease variants (single nucleotide polymorphisms, SNPs), have also recently identified potential susceptibility genes located on chromosome 2. These recent studies suggest a possible relationship between TS and obsessive-compulsive disorder (OCD)[199].

Although previous genetic studies have not identified genes that are definitely associated with the majority of TS cases, future studies will likely continue to search for rare mutations and more common genetic variations (polymorphisms). These studies will require very large sample sizes. The Tourette Association's International Genetic Consortium and the National Institutes of Health both continue to expand recruitment of subjects for genetic studies employing novel strategies[202]. These efforts are now joined by two additional groups: the Tourette International Collaborative Genetics (TIC Genetics) study involving many U.S., European and Asian countries, and the European Multicenter Tics in Children Studies (EMTICS), a consortium of tic disorder (TD) investigators in the European Union. In the months and years ahead, we are likely to see the development of collaborative efforts between these groups to share samples and perform cross-analyses of data in the search for the genes underlying TS and other TDs.

Environmental and lifestyle factors, perhaps acting in combination with genetic predispositions, have long been implicated in the development of TS[203, 204]. However, no specific factor, agent or lifestyle has been shown to play a role in TS. Studies are underway, notably in European countries where national healthcare registries are accessible, to determine if pre- and/or post-natal factors are associated with the development of TS[203-205]. There have also been unconfirmed reports of clustering of TS in some regions of the U.S., but these reports await larger analyses to determine the authenticity and if they are actual TS cases. Finally, there have been associations between TS and autoimmune disease[205], and though controversial, some cases may in the future be proven to have an antibody-mediated mechanism.

What have studies taught us about changes in the brain associated with Tourette?

The emergence, natural course and complex symptoms of TS suggest that it is actually a neurodevelopment disorder. However, the specific brain areas, networks and alterations underlying the condition remain unclear. Nevertheless, there are emerging clues that will require exploration in future studies.

Anatomical studies using imaging techniques have been recently performed in TS and point to alterations in the basal ganglia, cortex and other brain areas[206, 207]. In studies of subcortical regions, the results have been largely inconsistent with the exception of repeated observations of a decrease in the volume of an area of the brain called the caudate nucleus[208]. In contrast, cortical studies have demonstrated significant thinning of the frontal cortex and a decreased volume in other areas in TS as compared to control subjects[209]. These changes appear to develop in children and persist into adulthood. Diffusion tensor imaging (DTI) with or without transcranial magnetic stimulation (TMS) has provided some evidence for potential alterations in the structure and functions of the corpus callosum and motor cortex[210].

Functional MRI studies done on individuals with TS while performing motor or cognitive activities have revealed variations in cortical and subcortical regions when compared to control subjects[206]. Other studies have found cortical-subcortical network changes in adults with TS. The interpretation of these MRI findings is unclear, and they may relate to compensatory mechanisms in addition to or instead of causative changes.

Anatomical and functional studies, taken together, point to alterations of the cortico-striato-thalamo-cortical loops in the pathophysiology of TS. However, it is difficult to reconcile these emerging findings due in part to limited sample sizes, inconsistent population characteristics and different methodologies across studies. Some of these shortcomings are now being addressed by the Tourette Association of America Neuroimaging Consortium, a multi-center collaborative group examining structural MRI in a large, well-matched group of children and adolescents with and without TS. The first study from this group has shown increased gray matter volume in posterior thalamus, hypothalamus and midbrain, as well as lower white matter volumes in the orbital and medial prefrontal cortex[211]. These findings are consistent with reports in the literature of both subcortical and cortical changes in TS.

In future years, the TAA Neuroimaging Consortium and other groups will continue to explore other brain areas for alterations in TS using higher resolution equipment and better characterized samples[211]. Additionally, imaging protocols like these will require comparable protocols across different sites. There are also new and exciting avenues of study using neuroimaging techniques. For example, such studies might examine how the brains differ in individuals with different tic disorders and what brain changes are associated with the alterations in tic expression over time. It will be intriguing to determine the neuroimaging changes associated with the premonitory urge as this sensation precedes the actual tic in many pediatric and adult cases of TS. Finally, as we understand the genetics of TS better, it will be interesting to determine if different genetic subgroups are associated with different brain structures and functions. Finally, behavioral therapy, such as CBIT, has been recently shown to be effective in reducing tics[212]. It will be interesting to determine how this therapy actually alters brain networks.

What are some treatments on the horizon for Tourette?

The clinical features of TS can vary significantly within each individual over time and also among individuals with TS. The condition responds unpredictably to the various treatment options and may present with treatment failures and adverse effects[213]. Thus, there continues to be a great need to develop effective and safe treatment options for TS and other tic disorders. In recent years, we have seen promising results including medication, behavioral, surgical and other novel therapeutic approaches.

Medications Traditionally, pharmacological treatments for TS have been based on agents acting on the dopaminergic (e.g. D2 receptor antagonists such as haloperidol and aripiprazole) and alpha-adrenoceptor agonists (e.g. clonidine and guanfacine)[213]. Agents acting on other receptors and neuronal systems are being explored with the emergence of promising results that will need to be further developed.

D1 Receptor Antagonists There have been considerations that D1 receptor blockers might be effective in reducing tics and as well as associated with a lower incidence of adverse effects as compared to D2 antagonists. These studies are underway to determine the efficacy of ecopipam, a D1 receptor blocker, in adults with TS[110]. In the first multicenter, non-randomized, open-label study of 50 or 100 mg of ecopipam taken orally and daily over several weeks, it was found that a modest reduction in tic severity was accompanied by mild to moderate adverse effects. Based on these results, Psyadon Pharmaceuticals planned a follow-up randomized, double-blind, placebo-controlled study to evaluate the efficacy of ecopipam (clinicaltrial.gov identifier: NCT02102698).

Dopamine Release Blockers There has been long-standing interest in tetrabenazine and other drugs to reduce tics by blocking the release of dopamine. This class of drugs acts through interactions with the vesicular monoamine transport system[214, 215]. In recent years several compounds like valbenazine, which have a better pharmacokinetic profile, have been developed and are now undergoing clinical trials for several movement disorders including TS[215]. Neurocrine Biosciences is currently conducting clinical trials with a compound (NBI-98854) in children, adolescents and adults with TS (clinicaltrials.gov identifier: NCT02256475). Similarly, Auspex Pharmaceuticals is currently evaluating the safety, tolerability and efficacy of SD-809 (Deutetrabenazine) in patients with moderate to severe TS (clinicaltrials.gov identifier: NCT02674321). These novel tetrabenazine-like agents may prove to be more tolerable and could improve compliance in TS.

Behavioral Therapy Behavioral research and the development of therapies, notably CBIT, have collectively demonstrated remarkable progress over the past five years. Two clinical trials have been recently published and demonstrate the efficacy in both children and adults with TS[53, 54]. These studies have opened new avenues of research and development into behavioral therapies. Notably, the TAA and other organizations are now exploring and developing strategies to train more care providers in CBIT. Additionally, there is great interest in optimizing this new treatment strategy to facilitate the feasibility and adoption by other specialists including occupational therapists[216]. Additionally, work is underway to develop novel methods for CBIT via telemedicine and online portals. These efforts will have the combined effect of increasing patient access to behavioral therapies for tic and if successful could become a reasonable, accessible and feasible first line of treatment.

Deep Brain Stimulation DBS has been shown to be effective in reducing tics in select individuals with severe, drug-resistant TS[217]. In an effort to advance this treatment option, the TAA developed an international DBS registry and database to collect available data, such as lead targets and outcome measures, on all DBS procedures performed worldwide[129]. At present, the database has accumulated information from over 150 TS patients who underwent DBS procedures in 10 countries. The DBS Collaborative Study Group has published a consensus guideline on the use of DBS[129]. The registry will continue to serve as a focal point of collaboration and research, and it can be used to generate new data and drive the field toward regulatory approval for DBS in the U.S. and other countries. In addition, the group at the University of Florida has had several large federal grants to develop smart DBS techniques to sense tics in the brain before they occur and deliver an impulse to suppress them (closed loop DBS).

Dental Devices There has been considerable interest in dental orthotic devices as potential treatments for tic. Over the past few years, there have been numerous anecdotal reports and testimonials suggesting that these devices, which resemble traditional mouth guards used for TMJ, can reduce tic severity in individuals with TS. In responding to the needs of the community, the TAA recently commissioned and funded a double-blind, placebo-controlled, clinical trial to evaluate data on the safety and efficacy of the oral orthotic (clinicaltrials.gov identifier: NCT02067819). The primary aim of this study will be to evaluate feasibility of an active versus sham oral orthotic over two weeks. The study will assess whether it is feasible to reduce tic severity, and it will assess the durability of the effect over an additional four to six weeks. Secondary aims of this study will include assessing the safety, tolerability and initial efficacy of this device in reducing tic symptom severity.

Conclusions

Over the years, significant progress has been made across many areas of TS. However, there remain many unmet needs. For example, while TS is clearly hereditary, the specific genes and neurobiological changes underlying the development of the complex symptoms are unknown. Although care providers are better positioned to provide accurate and timely diagnoses of tics, there continues to be a need for effective, safe and reliable treatment options for affected individuals. Thus, there continues to be a need for active national and international research programs for TS. The TAA, ESSTS and other groups have embraced these challenges and are working to drive research and development in all areas of TS. It is expected that these efforts will be accelerated in the years ahead and will likely lead to significant advances in our understanding of and ability to manage TS and related disorders. We recommend you always ask your doctor the question: "What's new in TS therapy?"

⚘ Secret #10: Ask your doctor at every visit what's new in Tourette syndrome therapy.

Take Home Points:

- We are making important progress in understanding TS and have recently evolved to recognize this disorder as neurodevelopmental rather than neurodegenerative.

- There have been important advances in genetics and are several ongoing genetics consortia. The role of genetics in TS is likely complex as the disorder is highly heritable (genetic); however, few single-gene DNA defects have been uncovered.

- Imaging studies have identified changes in the brain's structure and function, and some of these imaging sequences may provide important biomarkers for future treatment trials.

- There are a number of drug, device and behavioral treatments in clinical trials, and these can be found at clinicaltrials.gov.

* * *

About the author:

Michael S. Okun, MD, was the author of the Amazon bestseller Parkinson's Treatment: 10 Secrets to a Happier Life which was translated into over 20 languages. His laboratory focuses on research underpinning Parkinson's, Tourette, and other movement disorders and he is active in the development of new treatments and devices. He was recently recognized at the White House as a Champion of Change for his work in these areas. Dr. Okun is currently Chairman of Neurology, Professor and Co-director of the 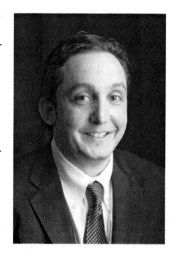 Center for Movement Disorders and Neurorestoration at the University of Florida College of Medicine. The center is unique in that it is comprised of 40+ interdisciplinary faculty members from diverse areas of campus, all of whom are dedicated to care, outreach, education and research. He was instrumental in the construction of a one-stop patient-centered clinical-research experience for national and international patients seen at the University of Florida. Dr. Okun is the Co-chair of the Medical Advisory Board for the Tourette Association of America and the National Medical Director for the Parkinson's Foundation. Dr. Okun has enjoyed a prolific research career exploring Tourette syndrome and non-motor basal ganglia brain features. He is currently developing a device to identify and treat tics through a NIH funded project. He has been an integral part of some of the pioneering studies exploring the cognitive, behavioral, and mood effects of brain stimulation. Dr. Okun holds the Adelaide Lackner Professorship in Neurology and has published over 350 peer-reviewed articles. He is a poet (Lessons From the Bedside, 1995) and his books on Parkinson's (Parkinson's Treatment: 10 Secrets to a Happier Life and 10 Breakthrough Therapies in Parkinson's Disease) have both been Amazon bestsellers.

* * *

References

1. Gunduz, A., Okun, M.S., A Review and Update on Tourette Syndrome: Where Is the Field Headed? Current Neurology and Neuroscience Reports 2016; 16:37.

2. Itard, J.M., Me′moire sur quelques functions involontaires des appareils de la locomotion, de la pre′hension et de la voix [French]. Arch Gen Med 1825; 8:385-407.

3. Trousseau, A., Clinique Me′dicale de l'Ho^tel Dieu de Paris Paris: J.-B. Bailliere, 1868.

4. Gilles de la Tourette G. Etude sur une affection nerveuse caracterisee par de l'incoordination morice accompagnee d'echoalie et de corolalie. Arch Neurol 1885; 9:158-200.

5. Albin, R.L., Mink, J.W., Recent Advances in Tourette Syndrome Research. Trends Neurosci 2006; 29:175-182.

6. Arzimanoglou, A.A. Gilles de la Tourette syndrome. J Neurol: Springer, 1998: 761-765.

7. Cavanna, A.E., Seri, S., Tourette's syndrome. BMJ2013: f4964.

8. State, M.W. The genetics of Tourette disorder. Current Opinion in Genetics & Development 2011.

9. Swain, J.E., Leckman, J.F., Tourette syndrome and tic disorders: overview and practical guide to diagnosis and treatment. Psychiatry (Edgmont) 2005; 2:26-36.

10. Tallur, K., Minns, R.A., Tourette's syndrome. Paediatrics and Child Health 2010; 20:88-93.

11. Thomas, R., Cavanna, A.E., The pharmacology of Tourette syndrome - Springer. Journal of Neural Transmission 2013.

12. Trivet, H.A., Chien, H.F., Munhoz, R.P., Barbosa, E.R., Charcot's contribution to the study of Tourette syndrome. Arq Neuropsiquiatr 2008; 66:918-921.

13. Leckman, J., Cohen, D., Tourette's Syndrome – Tics, Obsessions, Compulsions: Developmental Psychopathology and Clinical Care: John Wiley & Sons, 1999.

14. Leckman, J., Cohen, D.J., Goetz, C.G., Jankovic, J., Tourette Syndrome: Pieces of the Puzzle. Advances in Neurology 2001; 85.

15. Leckman, J., Peterson, B.S., Pauls, D., Cohen, D.J., Tic disorders. The Psychiatric Clinics of North America 1997; 20:839-861.

16. Leckman, J., Walker, D., Cohen, D., Premonitory urges in Tourette's syndrome. Am J Psychiatry 1993; 150.

17. Leckman, J.F., Tourette's syndrome. Lancet 2002; 360:1577-1586.

18. Freeman, R.D., Zinner, S.H., Muller-Vahl K.R., et al., Coprophenomena in Tourette syndrome. Developmental Medicine and Child Neurology 2009; 51:218-227.

19. Gilles de la Tourette G. E'tude sur une affection nerveuse caracte'rise'e par de l'incoordination motrice accompagne'e d'e'cholalie et de coprolalie [French]. Arch Neurol 1885; 9:158-200.

20. Gravino, G., Gilles de la Tourette syndrome. Ann Clin Psychiatry 2013: 297-306.

21. Hanna, P.A., Jankovic, J., Sleep and tic disorders. Woburn, MA: Butterworth-Heinemann, 2003.

22. Jankovic, J., Kurlan, R., Tourette syndrome: evolving concepts. Mov Disord 2011; 26:1149-1156.

23. Singer, H.S., Treatment of tics and tourette syndrome. Curr Treat Options Neurol 2010; 12:539-561.

24. American Physical Therapy A. Guide to Physical Therapist Practice. Second Edition. American Physical Therapy Association. Physical therapy 2001; 81:9-746.

25. Association AOT. American Occupational Therapy Association. (2014).Occupational therapy practice framework: Domain and process (3rd ed.). American Journal of Occupational Therapy 2014;68 (Suppl. 1):S1-S48.

26. Association APT. A Guide to Physical Therapy Practice 3.0. 2014.

27. Association AS-L-H. Learn About the CSD Professions: Speech-Language Pathology: Careers in Speech-Language Pathology. [online]. Available at: Available from http://www.asha.org/Students/Speech-Language-Pathology/

28. Bitsko, R.H., Holbrook, J.R., Visser, S.N., et al., A national profile of Tourette syndrome, 2011-2012. Journal of Developmental & Behavioral Pediatrics: JDBP 2014; 35:317-322.

29. Case-Smith, J., O'Brien, J. C., Occupational therapy for children: Elsevier Health Sciences, 2005.

30. Leckman, J.F., Bloch, M.H., Smith, M.E., Larabi, D., Hampson, M., Neurobiological substrates of Tourette's disorder. J Child Adolesc Psychopharmacol 2010; 20:237-247.

31. America TAo. Newly Diagnosed [online]. Available at: http://tourette. org/aPeople/Parents/parents.html.

32. America TAo. What is Tourette Syndrome? [online]. Available at: http://www.tourette.org/Medical/whatists_cov.html.

33. Occupational Therapy Practice Framework: Domain and Process. The American Journal of Occupational Therapy: official publication of the American Occupational Therapy Association 2002; 56:609-639.

34. Mahone, E.M., Cirino, P.T., Cutting, L.E., et al., Validity of the behavior rating inventory of executive function in children with ADHD and/or Tourette syndrome. Archives of Clinical Neuropsychology: the official journal of the National Academy of Neuropsychologists 2002; 17:643-662.

35. Singer, H.S., Tourette's syndrome: from behaviour to biology. Lancet Neurol 2005; 4:149-159.

36. Cox, J.H., Cavanna, A.E., Irritability symptoms in Gilles de la Tourette syndrome. The Journal of Neuropsychiatry and Clinical Neurosciences 2015; 27:42-47.

37. Chang, H.L., Liang, H.Y., Wang, H.S., Li, C.S., Ko, N.C., Hsu, Y.P., Behavioral and emotional problems in adolescents with Tourette syndrome. Chang Gung Medical Journal 2008; 31:145-152.

38. Reese, H.E., Vallejo, Z., Rasmussen, J., Crowe, K., Rosenfield, E., Wilhelm, S., Mindfulness-based stress reduction for Tourette Syndrome and Chronic Tic Disorder: a pilot study. Journal of Psychosomatic Research 2015; 78:293-298.

39. Michaels, E., Korman, C., Frank, G. Identification of Social Skills Deficits in Children with Tourette Syndrome (TS) [online]. Available at: http://tourette.org/pubsonline/A-128DD.pdf.

40. Rowe, J.M., Occupational Therapy & Speech-Language Pathology Services: What are they and how can they help? [online]. Available at: http://tourette.org/news/2014ConfPresentations/education_otspeech_malleyrowe.pdf

41. Farahmand, F., Abedi, A., Esmaeili-Dooki, M.R., Jalilian, R., Tabari, S.M., Pelvic Floor Muscle Exercise for Paediatric Functional Constipation. Journal of Clinical and Diagnostic Research: JCDR 2015; 9:SC16-17.

42. Comings, D.E., Comings, B.G., A controlled study of Tourette syndrome. VI. Early development, sleep problems, allergies, and handedness. American Journal of Human Genetics 1987; 41:822-838.

43. von Gontard, A., Equit, M., Comorbidity of ADHD and incontinence in children. European Child & Adolescent Psychiatry 2015; 24:127-140.

44. How much sleep do we actually need? [online]. Available at: https://sleepfoundation.org/how-sleep-works/how-much-sleep-do-we-really-need.

45. Ghosh, D., Rajan, P.V., Das, D., Datta, P., Rothner, A.D., Erenberg, G., Sleep disorders in children with Tourette syndrome. Pediatric Neurology 2014; 51:31-35.

46. Modafferi, S., Stornelli, M., Chiarotti, F., Cardona, F., Bruni, O., Sleep, anxiety and psychiatric symptoms in children with Tourette syndrome and tic disorders. European Journal of Paediatric Neurology: EJPN: official journal of the European Paediatric Neurology Society 2016;20:696-703.

47. Wadman, R., Tischler, V., Jackson, G. M., 'Everybody just thinks I'm weird': a qualitative exploration of the psychosocial experiences of adolescents with Tourette syndrome. Child: Care, Health and Development 2013; 39:880-886.

48. De Nil, L.F., Sasisekaran, J., Van Lieshout, P.H., Sandor, P., Speech disfluencies in individuals with Tourette syndrome. Journal of Psychosomatic Research 2005; 58:97-102.

49. Malley, P.W., Tourette Syndrome Education: Ask the Expert, Speech Therapy [online]. Available at: http://tourette.org/Education/Speech_Therapy.htm.

50. Liu, W.Y., Ya, T., Lien, H.Y., et al., Deficits in sensory organization for postural stability in children with Tourette syndrome. Clinical Neurology and Neurosurgery 2015; 129 Suppl 1:S36-40.

51. Nixon, E., Glazebrook, C., Hollis, C., Jackson, G.M., Reduced Tic Symptomatology in Tourette Syndrome After an Acute Bout of Exercise: An Observational Study. Behavior Modification 2014; 38:235-263.

52. Goodrich, B., Garza, E., The Role of Occupational Therapy in Providing Assistive Technology Devices and Services [online]. Available at: http://www.aota.org/About-Occupational-Therapy/Professionals/RDP/assistive-technology.aspx - sthash.CdNgyWpV.dpuf.

53. Piacentini, J., Woods, D.W., Scahill, L., et al., Behavior therapy for children with Tourette disorder: a randomized controlled trial. JAMA 2010; 303:1929-1937.

54. Wilhelm, S., Peterson, A.L., Piacentini, J.C., Woods, D.W., Deckersbach, T., Sukhodolsky, D.G., Chang, S., Liu, H., Dzuria, J., Walkup, J.T., Scahill, L., Randomized trial of behavior therapy for adults with Tourette's disorder. Archives of General Psychiatry 2012; 69:795-803.

55. Woods, D.W., Piacentini, J.C., Chang, S., Deckersbach, T., Ginsburg, G., Peterson, A.L., Scahill, L.D., Walkup, J.R., Wilhelm, S., Managing Tourette's Syndrome: A Behavioral Intervention

for Children and Adults (Therapist Guide). New York: Oxford University Press, 2008.

56. Woods, D.W., Piacentini, J.C., Scahill, L.D., Peterson, A.L., Wilhelm, S., Walkup, J.T., Behavior Therapy for Tics in Children: Acute and long term effects on secondary psychiatric and psychosocial functioning. Journal of Child Neurology 2011; 26:858-865.

57. Woods, D.W., Twohig, M.P., Flessner, C.A., Roloff, T.J., Treatment of vocal tics in children with Tourette syndrome: investigating the efficacy of habit reversal. Journal of Applied Behavior Analysis 2003; 36:109-112.

58. Dornbush, M.P., Pruitt, S.K., Tigers, Too: Executive Functions/ Speed of Processing/Memory: Impact on Academic, Behavioral, and Social Function of Students with ADHD, Tourette Syndrome and OCD: Modifications and Interventions, 1st ed. Atlanta, GA: Parkaire Press, Inc., 2009.

59. Taibbi, R., Doing Family Therapy, Second Edition: Craft and Creativity in Clinical Practice, 2nd Edition. New York: The Guilford Press, 2007.

60. Malaty, I.A., Akbar, U., Updates in medical and surgical therapies for Tourette syndrome. Current Neurology and Neuroscience Reports 2014; 14:458.

61. Freeman, R.D., Fast, D.K., Burd, L., Kerbeshian, J., Robertson, M.M., Sandor, P., An international perspective on Tourette syndrome: selected findings from 3,500 individuals in 22 countries. Developmental Medicine and Child Neurology 2000; 42:436-447.

62. Bloch, M.H., Peterson, B.S., Scahill, L., et al., Adulthood outcome of tic and obsessive-compulsive symptom severity in children with Tourette syndrome. Archives of Pediatrics & Adolescent Medicine 2006; 160:65-69.

63. Kraft, J.T., Dalsgaard, S., Obel, C., Thomsen, P.H., Henriksen, T.B., Scahill, L., Prevalence and clinical correlates of tic disorders in a community sample of school-age children. European Child & Adolescent Psychiatry 2012; 21:5-13.

64. Pringsheim, T., Doja, A., Gorman, D., et al., Canadian guidelines for the evidence-based treatment of tic disorders: pharmacotherapy. Canadian Journal of Psychiatry/ La Revue Canadienne de Psychiatrie 2012; 57:133-143.

65. Waldon, K., Hill, J., Termine, C., Balottin, U., Cavanna, A.E., Trials of pharmacological interventions for Tourette syndrome: a systematic review. Behavioural Neurology 2013; 26:265-273.

66. Roessner, V., Plessen, K.J., Rothenberger, A., et al., European clinical guidelines for Tourette syndrome and other tic disorders. Part II: pharmacological treatment. European Child & Adolescent Psychiatry 2011; 20:173-196.

67. Du, Y.S., Li, H.F., Vance, A., et al., Randomized double-blind multicentre placebo-controlled clinical trial of the clonidine adhesive patch for the treatment of tic disorders. The Australian and New Zealand Journal of Psychiatry 2008; 42:807-813.

68. Tourette's Syndrome Study Group, Treatment of ADHD in children with tics: a randomized controlled trial. Neurology 2002; 58:527-536.

69. Hartmann, A., Worbe, Y., Pharmacological treatment of Gilles de la Tourette syndrome. Neuroscience and Biobehavioral Reviews 2013; 37:1157-1161.

70. Boon-yasidhi, V., Kim, Y.S., Scahill, L., An open-label, prospective study of guanfacine in children with ADHD and tic disorders. Journal of the Medical Association of Thailand = Chotmaihet thangphaet 2005; 88 Suppl 8:S156-162.

71. Chappell, P.B., Riddle, M.A., Scahill, L., et al., Guanfacine treatment of comorbid attention-deficit hyperactivity disorder and

Tourette's syndrome: preliminary clinical experience. Journal of the American Academy of Child and Adolescent Psychiatry 1995; 34:1140-1146.

72. Cummings, D.D., Singer, H.S., Krieger, M., Miller, T.L., Mahone, E.M., Neuropsychiatric effects of guanfacine in children with mild tourette syndrome: a pilot study. Clinical Neuropharmacology 2002; 25:325-332.

73. Scahill, L., Chappell, P.B., Kim, Y.S., et al., A placebo-controlled study of guanfacine in the treatment of children with tic disorders and attention deficit hyperactivity disorder. Am J Psychiatry 2001; 158:1067-1074.

74. Shapiro, A.K., Shapiro, E., Treatment of Gilles de la Tourette's Syndrome with haloperidol. The British Journal of Psychiatry: the journal of mental science 1968; 114:345-350.

75. Shapiro, A.K., Shapiro, E., Wayne, H., Treatment of Tourette's syndrome with haloperidol, review of 34 cases. Arch Gen Psychiatry 1973; 28:92-97.

76. Muller-Vahl, K.R., Krueger, D., Does Tourette syndrome prevent tardive dyskinesia? Mov Disord 2011; 26:2442-2443.

77. Muller-Vahl, K.R., Roessner, V., Treatment of tics in patients with Tourette syndrome: recommendations according to the European Society for the Study of Tourette Syndrome. Mov Disord 2011; 26:2447; author reply 2448.

78. Wijemanne, S., Wu, L.J., Jankovic, J., Long-term efficacy and safety of fluphenazine in patients with Tourette syndrome. Mov Disord 2014; 29:126-130.

79. Cheng, W., Lin, L., Guo, S., [A Meta-analysis of the effectiveness of risperidone versus traditional agents for Tourette's syndrome]. Zhong nan da xue xue bao Yi xue ban = Journal of Central South University Medical Sciences 2012; 37:359-365.

80. Copur, M., Arpaci, B., Demir, T., Narin, H., Clinical effectiveness of quetiapine in children and adolescents with Tourette's syndrome : a retrospective case-note survey. Clinical Drug Investigation 2007; 27:123-130.

81. Mukaddes, N.M., Abali, O., Quetiapine treatment of children and adolescents with Tourette's disorder. Journal of Child and Adolescent Psychopharmacology 2003; 13:295-299.

82. Masi, G., Gagliano, A., Siracusano, R., et al., Aripiprazole in children with Tourette's disorder and co-morbid attention-deficit/hyperactivity disorder: a 12-week, open-label, preliminary study. Journal of Child and Adolescent Psychopharmacology 2012; 22:120-125.

83. Wenzel, C., Kleimann, A., Bokemeyer, S., Muller-Vahl, K.R., Aripiprazole for the treatment of Tourette syndrome: a case series of 100 patients. Journal of Clinical Psychopharmacology 2012; 32:548-550.

84. Yoo, H.K., Joung, Y.S., Lee, J.S., et al., A multicenter, randomized, double-blind, placebo-controlled study of aripiprazole in children and adolescents with Tourette's disorder. The Journal of Clinical Psychiatry 2013; 74:e772-780.

85. Liu, Z.S., Chen, Y.H., Zhong, Y.Q., et al., [A multicenter controlled study on aripiprazole treatment for children with Tourette syndrome in China]. Zhonghua er ke za zhi = Chinese Journal of Pediatrics 2011; 49:572-576.

86. Sallee, F.R., Kurlan, R., Goetz, C.G., et al., Ziprasidone treatment of children and adolescents with Tourette's syndrome: a pilot study. Journal of the American Academy of Child and Adolescent Psychiatry 2000; 39:292-299.

87. Kenney, C., Hunter, C., Jankovic, J., Long-term tolerability of tetrabenazine in the treatment of hyperkinetic movement disorders. Mov Disord 2007; 22:193-197.

88. Kenney, C., Jankovic, J., Tetrabenazine in the treatment of hyperkinetic movement disorders. Expert Review of Neurotherapeutics 2006; 6:7-17.

89. Porta, M., Sassi, M., Cavallazzi, M., Fornari, M., Brambilla, A., Servello, D., Tourette's syndrome and role of tetrabenazine: review and personal experience. Clinical Drug Investigation 2008; 28:443-459.

90. Mehanna, R., Hunter, C., Davidson, A., Jimenez-Shahed, J., Jankovic, J., Analysis of CYP2D6 genotype and response to tetrabenazine. Mov Disord 2013; 28:210-215.

91. Ondo, W.G., Jong, D., Davis, A., Comparison of weight gain in treatments for Tourette syndrome: tetrabenazine versus neuroleptic drugs. Journal of Child Neurology 2008; 23:435-437.

92. Yang, C.S., Zhang, L.L., Zeng, L.N., Huang, L., Liu, Y.T., Topiramate for Tourette's syndrome in children: a meta-analysis. Pediatric Neurology 2013; 49:344-350.

93. Jankovic, J., Jimenez-Shahed, J., Brown, L.W., A randomised, double-blind, placebo-controlled study of topiramate in the treatment of Tourette syndrome. Journal of Neurology, Neurosurgery, and Psychiatry 2010; 81:70-73.

94. Gonce, M., Barbeau, A., Seven cases of Gilles de la tourette's syndrome: partial relief with clonazepam: a pilot study. The Canadian Journal of Neurological Sciences/Le Journal Canadien des Sciences Neurologiques 1977; 4:279-283.

95. Kaim, B., A case of Gilles de la Tourette's syndrome treated with clonazepam. Brain Research Bulletin 1983; 11:213-214.

96. Merikangas, J.R., Merikangas, K.R., Kopp, U., Hanin, I., Blood choline and response to clonazepam and haloperidol in Tourette's syndrome. Acta Psychiatrica Scandinavica 1985; 72:395-399.

97. Awaad, Y., Tics in Tourette syndrome: new treatment options. Journal of Child Neurology 1999; 14:316-319.

98. Singer, H.S., Wendlandt, J., Krieger, M., Giuliano, J., Baclofen treatment in Tourette syndrome: a double-blind, placebo-controlled, crossover trial. Neurology 2001; 56:599-604.

99. Kwak, C.H., Hanna, P.A., Jankovic, J., Botulinum toxin in the treatment of tics. Archives of Neurology 2000; 57:1190-1193.

100. Marras, C., Andrews, D., Sime, E., Lang, A.E., Botulinum toxin for simple motor tics: a randomized, double-blind, controlled clinical trial. Neurology 2001; 56:605-610.

101. Porta, M., Maggioni, G., Ottaviani, F., Schindler, A., Treatment of phonic tics in patients with Tourette's syndrome using botulinum toxin type A. Neurological Sciences: official journal of the Italian Neurological Society and of the Italian Society of Clinical Neurophysiology 2004; 24:420-423.

102. Scott, B.L., Jankovic, J., Donovan, D.T., Botulinum toxin injection into vocal cord in the treatment of malignant coprolalia associated with Tourette's syndrome. Mov Disord 1996; 11:431-433.

103. Anca, M.H., Giladi, N., Korczyn, A.D., Ropinirole in Gilles de la Tourette syndrome. Neurology 2004; 62:1626-1627.

104. Gilbert, D.L., Dure, L., Sethuraman, G., Raab, D., Lane, J., Sallee, F.R., Tic reduction with pergolide in a randomized controlled trial in children. Neurology 2003; 60:606-611.

105. Gilbert, D.L., Sethuraman, G., Sine, L., Peters, S., Sallee, F.R., Tourette's syndrome improvement with pergolide in a randomized, double-blind, crossover trial. Neurology 2000; 54:1310-1315.

106. Kurlan, R., Crespi, G., Coffey, B., et al., A multicenter randomized placebo-controlled clinical trial of pramipexole for Tourette's syndrome. Mov Disord 2012; 27:775-778.

107. McConville, B.J., Sanberg, P.R., Fogelson, M.H., et al., The effects of nicotine plus haloperidol compared to nicotine only and placebo nicotine only in reducing tic severity and frequency in Tourette's disorder. Biol Psychiatry 1992; 31:832-840.

108. Silver, A.A., Shytle, R.D., Philipp, M.K., Wilkinson, B.J., McConville, B., Sanberg, P.R. Transdermal nicotine and haloperidol in Tourette's disorder: a double-blind placebo-controlled study. The Journal of Clinical Psychiatry 2001; 62:707-714.

109. Howson, A.L., Batth, S., Ilivitsky, V., et al., Clinical and attentional effects of acute nicotine treatment in Tourette's syndrome. European Psychiatry: the journal of the Association of European Psychiatrists 2004; 19:102-112.

110. Gilbert, D.L., Budman, C.L., Singer, H.S., Kurlan, R., Chipkin, R.E., A D1 receptor antagonist, ecopipam, for treatment of tics in Tourette syndrome. Clinical Neuropharmacology 2014; 37:26-30.

111. Benabid, A.L., What the future holds for deep brain stimulation. Expert Rev Med Devices 2007; 4:895-903.

112. Benabid, A.L., Benazzouz, A., Hoffmann, D., Limousin, P., Krack, P., Pollak, P., Long-Term Electrical Inhibition of Deep Brain Targets in Movement Disorders. Movement Disorders 1998; 13:119-125.

113. Benabid, A.L., Chabardes, S., Torres, N., et al., Functional neurosurgery for movement disorders: a historical perspective. Prog Brain Res 2009; 175:379-391.

114. Benabid, A.L., Koudsie, A., Benazzouz, A., et al., Subthalamic stimulation for Parkinson's disease. Arch Med Res 2000; 31:282-289.

115. Benabid, A.L., Koudsie, A., Benazzouz, A., et al., Deep brain stimulation of the corpus luysi (subthalamic nucleus) and other targets in Parkinson's disease. Extension to new indications such as dystonia and epilepsy. J Neurol 2001; 248 Suppl 3:III37-47.

116. Benabid, A.L., Pollak, P., Louveau, A., Henry, S., de Rougemont, J., Combined (thalamotomy and stimulation) stereotactic surgery of the VIM thalamic nucleus for bilateral Parkinson disease. Appl Neurophysiol 1987; 50:344-346.

117. Benabid, A.L., Pollak, P., Seigneuret, E., Hoffmann, D., Gay, E., Perret, J. Chronic VIM thalamic stimulation in Parkinson's disease, essential tremor and extra-pyramidal dyskinesias. Acta Neurochir Suppl (Wien) 1993; 58:39-44.

118. Okun, M.S., Parkinson's Treatment: 10 Secrets to a Happier Life: Books4Patients, 2013.

119. de Hemptinne, C., Ryapolova-Webb, E.S., Air, E.L., et al., Exaggerated phase-amplitude coupling in the primary motor cortex in Parkinson disease. Proceedings of the National Academy of Sciences of the United States of America 2013; 110:4780-4785.

120. Shute, J., Maling, N., Rossi, P.J., et al., Neural correlates of Tourette syndrome within the centromedian thalamus, premotor and primary motor cortices. Neuroscience Annual Meeting; 2014; Washington, DC.

121. Okun, M.S., Foote, K.D., A mnemonic for Parkinson disease patients considering DBS: a tool to improve perceived outcome of surgery. Neurologist 2004; 10:290.

122. Okun, M.S., Fernandez, H.H., Rodriguez, R.L., Foote, K.D., Identifying candidates for deep brain stimulation in Parkinson's disease: the role of the primary care physician. Geriatrics 2007; 62:18-24.

123. Okun, M.S., Fernandez, H.H., Pedraza, O., et al., Development and initial validation of a screening tool for Parkinson disease surgical candidates. Neurology 2004; 63:161-163.

124. Okun, M.S., Deep-brain stimulation for Parkinson's disease. N Engl J Med 2012; 367:1529-1538.

125. Gunduz, A., Morita, H., Rossi, P.J., et al., Proceedings of the Second Annual Deep Brain Stimulation Think Tank: What's in the Pipeline. The International Journal of Neuroscience 2015; 125:475-485.

126. Schrock, L.E., Mink, J.W., Woods, D.W., et al., Tourette syndrome deep brain stimulation: A review and updated recommendations. Mov Disord 2015; 40:448-471.

127. Rossi, P.J., Gunduz, A., Judy, J., et al., Proceedings of the Third Annual Deep Brain Stimulation Think Tank: A Review of Emerging Issues and Technologies. Frontiers in Neuroscience 2016; 10:119.

128. Almeida, L., Martinez-Ramirez, D., Rossi, P.J., Peng, Z., Gunduz, A., Okun, M.S., Chasing tics in the human brain: development of open, scheduled and closed loop responsive approaches to deep brain stimulation for tourette syndrome. Journal of Clinical Neurology 2015; 11:122-131.

129. Deeb, W., Rossi, P.J., Porta, M., et al., The International Deep Brain Stimulation Registry and Database for Gilles de la Tourette Syndrome: How Does It Work? Frontiers in Neuroscience 2016; 10:170.

130. Rossi, P.J., Giordano, J., Okun, M.S., The Problem of Funding Off-label Deep Brain Stimulation: Bait-and-Switch Tactics and the Need for Policy Reform. JAMA Neurol 2016.

131. Baldwin, B., The career and work of Scribonius Largus. Rheinisches Museum Für Philologie 1992; 135:74-82.

132. Goetz, C.G., Chmura, T.A., Lanska, D.J., History of tic disorders and Gilles de la Tourette syndrome: part 5 of the MDS-sponsored history of movement disorders exhibit, Barcelona, June 2000. Mov Disord 2001; 16:346-349.

133. Girard, P.F., Les tics. Traité de Médecine 1949; 16:1183-1190.

134. Kushner, H.I., A cursing brain?: the histories of Tourette syndrome. Cambridge, Mass. Harvard University Press, 1999.

135. Swerdlow, N.R., Gierz, M., Berkowitz, A., Nemiroff, R., Lohr, J., Electroconvulsive therapy in a patient with severe tic and major depressive episode. The Journal of Clinical Psychiatry 1990; 51:34-35.

136. Rapoport, M., Feder, V., Sandor, P., Response of major depression and Tourette's syndrome to ECT: a case report. Psychosomatic Medicine 1998; 60:528-529.

137. Rajashree, V.C., Manjiri, C.D., Ivan, S.N., Alka, V.P., Gilles de la Tourette's syndrome successfully treated with electroconvulsive therapy. Indian Journal of Psychiatry 2014; 56:407-408.

138. Guttmacher, L.B., Cretella, H., Electroconvulsive therapy in one child and three adolescents. The Journal of Clinical Psychiatry 1988; 49:20-23.

139. Garvey, M.A., Kaczynski, K.J., Becker, D.A., Bartko, J.J., Subjective reactions of children to single-pulse transcranial magnetic stimulation. Journal of Child Neurology 2001; 16:891-894.

140. Rossi, S., Hallett, M., Rossini, P.M., Pascual-Leone, A., Safety, ethical considerations, and application guidelines for the use of transcranial magnetic stimulation in clinical practice and research. Clin Neurophysiol 2009; 120:2008-2039.

141. Wassermann, E.M., Risk and safety of repetitive transcranial magnetic stimulation: report and suggested guidelines from the International Workshop on the Safety of Repetitive Transcranial Magnetic Stimulation, June 5-7, 1996. Electroencephalogr Clin Neurophysiol 1998; 108:1-16.

142. Hong, Y.H., Wu, S.W., Pedapati, E.V., et al., Safety and tolerability of theta burst stimulation vs. single and paired pulse transcranial magnetic stimulation: a comparative study of 165 pediatric subjects. Frontiers in Human Neuroscience 2015; 9:29.

143. Oberman, L., Edwards, D., Eldaief, M., Pascual-Leone, A., Safety of theta burst transcranial magnetic stimulation: a systematic review of the literature. J Clin Neurophysiol 2011; 28:67-74.

144. Krishnan, C., Santos, L., Peterson, M.D., Ehinger, M., Safety of Noninvasive Brain Stimulation in Children and Adolescents. Brain Stimul 2014.

145. Orth, M., Munchau, A., Rothwell, J.C., Corticospinal system excitability at rest is associated with tic severity in tourette syndrome. Biol Psychiatry 2008; 64:248-251.

146. Heise, K.F., Steven, B., Liuzzi, G., et al., Altered modulation of intracortical excitability during movement preparation in Gilles de la Tourette syndrome. Brain 2010; 133:580-590.

147. Draper, A., Jude, L., Jackson, G.M., Jackson, S.R., Motor excitability during movement preparation in Tourette syndrome. Journal of Neuropsychology 2013.

148. Jackson, S.R., Parkinson, A., Manfredi, V., Millon, G., Hollis, C., Jackson, G.M., Motor excitability is reduced prior to voluntary movements in children and adolescents with Tourette syndrome. Journal of Neuropsychology 2013; 7:29-44.

149. Kasai, T., Kawai, S., Kawanishi, M., Yahagi, S., Evidence for facilitation of motor evoked potentials (MEPs) induced by motor imagery. Brain Research 1997; 744:147-150.

150. Majid, D.S., Lewis, C., Aron, A.R., Training voluntary motor suppression with real-time feedback of motor evoked potentials. Journal of Neurophysiology 2015; 113:3446-3452.

151. Ziemann, U., Paulus, W., Rothenberger, A., Decreased motor inhibition in Tourette's disorder: evidence from transcranial magnetic stimulation. Am J Psychiatry 1997; 154:1277-1284.

152. Orth, M., Amann, B., Robertson, M.M., Rothwell, J.C., Excitability of motor cortex inhibitory circuits in Tourette syndrome before and after single dose nicotine. Brain 2005; 128:1292-1300.

153. Gilbert, D.L., Bansal, A.S., Sethuraman, G., et al., Association of cortical disinhibition with tic, ADHD, and OCD severity in Tourette syndrome. Mov Disord 2004; 19:416-425.

154. Moll, G.H., Heinrich, H., Trott, G.E., Wirth, S., Bock, N., Rothenberger, A., Children with comorbid attention-deficit-hyperactivity disorder and tic disorder: evidence for additive inhibitory deficits within the motor system. Annals of Neurology 2001; 49:393-396.

155. Goetz, C.G., Clonidine and clonazepam in Tourette syndrome. Advances in Neurology 1992; 58:245-251.

156. Wu, S.W., Gilbert, D.L., Altered neurophysiologic response to intermittent theta burst stimulation in Tourette syndrome. Brain Stimul 2012; 5:315-319.

157. Suppa, A., Belvisi, D., Bologna, M., et al., Abnormal cortical and brain stem plasticity in Gilles de la Tourette syndrome. Mov Disord 2011; 26:1703-1710.

158. Suppa, A., Marsili, L., Di Stasio, F., et al., Cortical and brainstem plasticity in Tourette syndrome and obsessive-compulsive disorder. Mov Disord 2014.

159. Brandt, V.C., Niessen, E., Ganos, C., Kahl, U., Baumer, T., Munchau, A., Altered synaptic plasticity in Tourette's syndrome and its relationship to motor skill learning. PloS one 2014; 9:e98417.

160. Martin-Rodriguez, J.F., Ruiz-Rodriguez, M.A., Palomar, F.J., et al., Aberrant cortical associative plasticity associated with severe adult Tourette syndrome. Mov Disord 2015; 30:431-435.

161. Scahill, L., Erenberg, G., Berlin, C.M., Jr., et al., Contemporary assessment and pharmacotherapy of Tourette syndrome. NeuroRx 2006; 3:192-206.

162. Karp, B.I., Wassermann, E.M., Porter, S., Hallett, M., Transcranial magnetic stimulation acutely decreases motor tics. Neurology 1997; 48:A397.

163. Munchau, A., Bloem, B.R., Thilo, K.V., Trimble, M.R., Rothwell, J.C., Robertson, M.M., Repetitive transcranial magnetic stimulation for Tourette syndrome. Neurology 2002; 59:1789-1791.

164. Orth, M., Kirby, R., Richardson, M.P., et al., Subthreshold rTMS over pre-motor cortex has no effect on tics in patients with Gilles de la Tourette syndrome. Clin Neurophysiol 2005; 116:764-768.

165. Chae, J.H., Nahas, Z., Wassermann, E., et al., A pilot safety study of repetitive transcranial magnetic stimulation (rTMS) in Tourette's syndrome. Cogn Behav Neurol 2004; 17:109-117.

166. Wu, S.W., Maloney, T., Gilbert, D.L., et al., Functional MRI-navigated repetitive transcranial magnetic stimulation over supplementary motor area in chronic tic disorders. Brain Stimul 2014; 7:212-218.

167. Mantovani, A., Leckman, J.F., Grantz, H., King, R.A., Sporn, A.L., Lisanby, S.H., Repetitive Transcranial Magnetic Stimulation of the Supplementary Motor Area in the treatment of Tourette Syndrome: report of two cases. Clin Neurophysiol 2007; 118:2314-2315.

168. Mantovani, A., Lisanby, S.H., Pieraccini, F., Ulivelli, M., Castrogiovanni, P., Rossi, S., Repetitive transcranial magnetic stimulation (rTMS) in the treatment of obsessive-compulsive disorder (OCD) and Tourette's syndrome (TS). Int J Neuropsychopharmacol 2006; 9:95-100.

169. Landeros-Weisenberger, A., Mantovani, A., Motlagh, M.G., et al., Randomized Sham Controlled Double-blind Trial of Repetitive Transcranial Magnetic Stimulation for Adults With Severe Tourette Syndrome. Brain Stimul 2015; 8:574-581.

170. Le, K., Liu, L., Sun, M., Hu, L., Xiao, N., Transcranial magnetic stimulation at 1 Hertz improves clinical symptoms in children with Tourette syndrome for at least 6 months. Journal of Clinical Neuroscience: official journal of the Neurosurgical Society of Australasia 2013; 20:257-262.

171. Kwon, H.J., Lim, W.S., Lim, M.H., et al., 1-Hz low frequency repetitive transcranial magnetic stimulation in children with Tourette's syndrome. Neuroscience Letters 2011; 492:1-4.

172. Ekici, B., Transcranial direct current stimulation-induced seizure: analysis of a case. Clinical EEG and Neuroscience 2015; 46:169.

173. Mrakic-Sposta, S., Marceglia, S., Mameli, F., Dilena, R., Tadini, L., Priori, A., Transcranial direct current stimulation in two patients with Tourette syndrome. Mov Disord 2008; 23:2259-2261.

174. Swedo, S.E., Leonard, H.L., Garvey, M., et al., Pediatric autoimmune neuropsychiatric disorders associated with streptococcal infections: clinical description of the first 50 cases. American Journal of Psychiatry 1998.

175. Ben-Pazi, H., Stoner, J.A., Cunningham, M.W., Dopamine receptor autoantibodies correlate with symptoms in Sydenham's chorea. PLOS ONE 2013; 8:e73516.

176. Chang, K., Frankovich, J., Cooperstock, M., et al., Clinical evaluation of youth with pediatric acute-onset neuropsychiatric syndrome (PANS): recommendations from the 2013 PANS Consensus Conference. Journal of Child and Adolescent Psychopharmacology 2015; 25:3-13.

177. Bitsko, R.H., Holbrook, J.R., Visser, S.N., et al., A national profile of Tourette syndrome, 2011–2012. Journal of Developmental and Behavioral Pediatrics: JDBP 2014; 35:317.

178. Singer, H.S., Giuliano, J.D., Zimmerman, A.M., Walkup, J.T., Infection: a stimulus for tic disorders. Pediatric Neurology 2000; 22:380-383.

179. Murphy, T.K., Lewin, A.B., Parker-Athill, E.C., Storch, E.A., Mutch, P.J., Tonsillectomies and adenoidectomies do not prevent the onset of pediatric autoimmune neuropsychiatric disorder associated with group A streptococcus. The Pediatric Infectious Disease Journal 2013; 32:834.

180. Murphy, T.K., Storch, E., Turner, A., Reid, J., Tan, J., Lewin, A., Maternal history of autoimmune disease in children presenting with tics and/or obsessive–compulsive disorder. Journal of Neuroimmunology 2010; 229:243-247.

181. Dalsgaard, S., Waltoft, B.L., Leckman, J.F., Mortensen, P.B., Maternal History of Autoimmune Disease and Later Development of Tourette Syndrome in Offspring. Journal of the American Academy of Child & Adolescent Psychiatry 2015; 54:495-501. e491.

182. Bernstein, G.A., Victor, A.M., Pipal, A.J., Williams, K.A., Comparison of clinical characteristics of pediatric autoimmune neuropsychiatric disorders associated with streptococcal infections and childhood obsessive-compulsive disorder. Journal of Child and Adolescent Psychopharmacology 2010; 20:333-340.

183. Murphy, T.K., Storch, E.A., Lewin, A.B., Edge, P.J., Goodman, W.K., Clinical factors associated with pediatric autoimmune neuropsychiatric disorders associated with streptococcal infections. The Journal of Pediatrics 2012; 160:314-319.

184. Snider, L.A., Lougee, L., Slattery, M., Grant, P., Swedo, S.E., Antibiotic prophylaxis with azithromycin or penicillin for

childhood-onset neuropsychiatric disorders. Biological Psychiatry 2005; 57:788-792.

185. Perlmutter, S.J., Leitman, S.F., Garvey, M.A., et al., Therapeutic plasma exchange and intravenous immunoglobulin for obsessive-compulsive disorder and tic disorders in childhood. The Lancet 1999; 354:1153-1158.

186. Williams, K.A., Swedo, S.E., Farmer, C.A., et al., Randomized, Controlled Trial of Intravenous Immunoglobulin for Pediatric Autoimmune Neuropsychiatric Disorders Associated With Streptococcal Infections. Journal of the American Academy of Child & Adolescent Psychiatry 2016; 55:860-867. e862.

187. Demesh, D., Virbalas, J.M., Bent, J.P., The role of tonsillectomy in the treatment of pediatric autoimmune neuropsychiatric disorders associated with streptococcal infections (PANDAS). JAMA Otolaryngology–Head & Neck Surgery 2015; 141:272-275.

188. Tona, J.P., Posner, T., Pediatric Autoimmune Neuropsychiatric Disorders: A New Frontier for Occupational Therapy Intervention. American Occupational Therapy Association OT Practice 2011.

189. Murphy, T.K., Kurlan, R., Leckman, J., The immunobiology of Tourette's disorder, pediatric autoimmune neuropsychiatric disorders associated with Streptococcus, and related disorders: a way forward. Journal of Child and Adolescent Psychopharmacology 2010; 20:317-331.

190. Murphy, T.K., Patel, P.D., McGuire, J.F., et al., Characterization of the pediatric acute-onset neuropsychiatric syndrome phenotype. Journal of Child and Adolescent Psychopharmacology 2015; 25:14-25.

191. Muller-Vahl, K.R., Cannabinoids reduce symptoms of Tourette's syndrome. Expert Opinion on Pharmacotherapy 2003; 4:1717-1725.

192. Muller-Vahl, K.R., Treatment of Tourette syndrome with cannabinoids. Behavioural Neurology 2013; 27:119-124.

193. Koppel, B.S., Brust, J.C., Fife, T., et al., Systematic review: efficacy and safety of medical marijuana in selected neurologic disorders: report of the Guideline Development Subcommittee of the American Academy of Neurology. Neurology 2014; 82:1556-1563.

194. Curtis, A., Clarke, C.E., Rickards, H.E., Cannabinoids for Tourette's Syndrome. The Cochrane database of systematic reviews 2009: CD006565.

195. Volkow, N.D., Baler, R.D., Compton, W.M., Weiss, S.R., Adverse health effects of marijuana use. The New England Journal of Medicine 2014; 370:2219-2227.

196. Okun, M.S., 10 Breakthrough Therapies for Parkinson's Disease: Books4Patients, 2015.

197. Diagnostic and Statistical manual of Mental Disorders, DSM-5. Washington, DC: American Psychiatric Publishing, 2013.

198. McNaught, K.S., Mink, J.W., Advances in understanding and treatment of Tourette syndrome. Nat Rev Neurol 2011; 7:667-676.

199. Scharf, J.M., Yu, D., Mathews, C.A., et al., Genome-wide association study of Tourette's syndrome. Molecular Psychiatry 2013; 18:721-728.

200. Ercan-Sencicek, A.G., Stillman, A.A., Ghosh, A.K., et al., L-histidine decarboxylase and Tourette's syndrome. The New England Journal of Medicine 2010; 362:1901-1908.

201. McGrath, L.M., Yu, D., Marshall, C., et al., Copy number variation in obsessive-compulsive disorder and tourette syndrome: a cross-disorder study. Journal of the American Academy of Child and Adolescent Psychiatry 2014; 53:910-919.

202. Egan, C.A., Marakovitz, S.E., O'Rourke, J.A., et al., Effectiveness of a web-based protocol for the screening and phenotyping of

individuals with Tourette syndrome for genetic studies. Am J Med Genet B Neuropsychiatr Genet 2012; 159B:987-996.

203. Ben-Shlomo, Y., Scharf, J.M., Miller, L.L., Mathews, C.A., Parental mood during pregnancy and post-natally is associated with offspring risk of Tourette syndrome or chronic tics: prospective data from the Avon Longitudinal Study of Parents and Children (ALSPAC). European Child & Adolescent Psychiatry 2016; 25:373-381.

204. Mathews, C.A., Scharf, J.M., Miller, L.L., Macdonald-Wallis, C., Lawlor, D.A., Ben-Shlomo, Y., Association between pre- and perinatal exposures and Tourette syndrome or chronic tic disorder in the ALSPAC cohort. The British Journal of Psychiatry: the Journal of Mental Science 2014; 204:40-45.

205. Mataix-Cols, D., Isomura, K., Perez-Vigil, A., et al., Familial Risks of Tourette Syndrome and Chronic Tic Disorders. A Population-Based Cohort Study. JAMA Psychiatry 2015; 72:787-793.

206. Church, J.A., Schlaggar, B.L., Pediatric Tourette syndrome: insights from recent neuroimaging studies. J Obsessive Compuls Relat Disord 2014; 3:386-393.

207. Plessen, K.J., Bansal, R., Peterson, B.S., Imaging evidence for anatomical disturbances and neuroplastic compensation in persons with Tourette syndrome. Journal of Psychosomatic Research 2009; 67:559-573.

208. Peterson, B.S., Thomas, P., Kane, M.J., et al., Basal Ganglia volumes in patients with Gilles de la Tourette syndrome. Arch Gen Psychiatry 2003; 60:415-424.

209. Sowell, E.R., Kan, E., Yoshii, J., et al., Thinning of sensorimotor cortices in children with Tourette syndrome. Nat Neurosci 2008; 11:637-639.

210. Cavanna, A.E., Stecco, A., Rickards, H., et al., Corpus callosum abnormalities in Tourette syndrome: an MRI-DTI study of

monozygotic twins. Journal of Neurology, Neurosurgery, and Psychiatry 2010; 81:533-535.

211. Green, D.J., Williams, A.C., Koller, J.M., Schlaggar, B.L., Black, K.J., and the Tourette Association of America Neuroimaging Consortium. Brain structure in pediatric Tourette syndrome. Molecular Psychiatry. Oct. 25, 2016.

212. Piacentini, J.C., Woods, D.W., Scahill, L.D., Wilhelm, S., Peterson, A., Chang, S., Ginsburg, G., Deckersbach, T., Dzuria, J., Levi-Pearl, S. & Walkup, J.T., Behavior Therapy for Children with Tourette Syndrome: A Randomized Controlled Trial. Journal of the American Medical Association 2010; 303:1929-1937.

213. Egolf, A., Coffey, B.J., Current pharmacotherapeutic approaches for the treatment of Tourette syndrome. Drugs Today (Barc) 2014; 50:159-179.

214. Muller, T., Valbenazine granted breakthrough drug status for treating tardive dyskinesia. Expert Opinion on Investigational Drugs 2015; 24:737-742.

215. O'Brien, C.F., Jimenez, R., Hauser, R.A., et al., NBI-98854, a selective monoamine transport inhibitor for the treatment of tardive dyskinesia: A randomized, double-blind, placebo-controlled study. Mov Disord 2015; 30:1681-1687.

216. Ricketts, E.J., Gilbert, D.L., Zinner, S.H., et al., Pilot Testing Behavior Therapy for Chronic Tic Disorders in Neurology and Developmental Pediatrics Clinics. Journal of Child Neurology 2016; 31:444-450.

217. Schrock, L.E., Mink, J.W., Woods, D.W., et al., Tourette syndrome deep brain stimulation: a review and updated recommendations. Mov Disord 2015; 30:448-471.

* * *

CPSIA information can be obtained
at www.ICGtesting.com
Printed in the USA
FSOW02n0858100417
32937FS

9 781542 484213